The Smoker's Guide to Vitamins and Health

Alistair D. Moodie B.S.

Vanguard Books Inc
Crofton
Maryland

Before beginning this or any other medical or nutritional regimen, consult your physician to be sure it is appropriate for you.
The author and publisher of this book are not physicians and are not licensed to give medical advice. All the information in this book came from clinical journals, scientific publications, medical journals, personal interviews, published books, magazine articles and self-published materials by experts. Any questions regarding your individual health, general or specific, should be addressed to your physician. The author and publisher disclaim any liability arising directly or indirectly from the use of this book.

Published by: Vanguard Books Inc
PO Box 4028
Crofton
MD 21114

Printed in the United States of America.

Cataloging in Publication Data
Moodie, Alistair D.
        The smoker's guide to vitamins and health: how to reduce the risks of smoking and protect your health
    Includes bibliographical references and index
1. Smoking   2. Health
3. Vitamins   4. Nutrition
ISBN 0-9647165-4-2
613.85   HV5740   LCCCN 95-061131

Dedication

This book is dedicated to my late father David Moodie MRCVS, DVSM, Scottish country veterinarian. He taught me how to think and instilled in me what commonsense I have. Standing on his shoulders I am able to write this book.

Praise is also due to my long-suffering wife Margaret, without her encouagement and infinite patience this book would never have reached the printers.

Acknowledgements

My thanks go out to my reviewers who despite very busy schedules, gave generously of their time to read and comment on this work. Their helpful suggestions and the material they provided were always of great value. They are: Robert A. Jacob, PhD, FACN, Hans-Anton Lehr, MD, PhD, Gladys Block, PhD, Harinder Garewal, MD, PhD, John H. Weisburger, PhD, MD (hon), FACN, James McD Robertson, DVM, MSc(Med).

Special thanks are due also to Professor Paul Lachance, Department of Food Science at Rutgers University for the many hours he spent correcting and commenting on the work and for all the background information he provided.

Kevin Kallaugher, better known as "Kal", political cartoonist for the Baltimore Sun, provided the cartoons which give some light relief to a serious subject.

Mention must also be made of the many scientists whose names appear only in the reference section. It is their unsung work in research centers and laboratories around the world which laid the foundations of knowledge from which this book was produced. I hope the book does justice to their work and will be of benefit to smokers.

Finally a word of thanks to the librarians and staff of the McKeldin Library, University of Maryland, at College Park. They were always helpful and patient in answering my many questions about their excellent collection of research material.

CONTENTS

Forewords

Gladys Block PhD,
Professor of Public Health and Nutrition,
University of California at Berkeley.

Recommending dietary changes for smokers is controversial. Everyone agrees that the best thing they can do for their health is to stop smoking. And so do I. But what about the person who has stopped, but is still at increased risk? And what about the person who is exposed to second-hand smoke? And what about the smoker who has tried to stop but has not yet been successful? If there is anything they can do to reduce their health risk, they have a right to know about it.

There is a great deal of research on the harmful effects of cigarette smoking (not just lung cancer!). But many people are not aware that there is also a great deal of research on fruits and vegetables and the antioxidant nutrients they provide, and how much they may reduce people's risk of harmful effects like heart disease and cancer. It is also known that smoking lowers blood levels of these antioxidants, and the National Academy of Sciences' Food and Nutrition Board has even set a higher daily requirement for vitamin C in smokers.

Alistair Moodie's book is a very well-researched and accurate summary of that research on smoking, vitamins and health. It will show you why you should get enough vitamins and fruits and vegetables, to reduce the harmful effects of cigarette smoke. Just as important he has very practical and specific suggestions about how to increase your intake of these nutrients. Even with today's busy lifestyles, it is possible to take valuable steps to protect your health.

Robert A. Jacob, PhD, FACN,
Research Chemist, Micronutrients Unit,
USDA Agricultural Research Service,
Western Human Nutrition Research Center,
Presidio of San Francisco, California.

Research studies have consistently shown that eating diets high in fruits and vegetables reduces the risk of developing many degenerative diseases, such as cancer, heart disease and eye cataracts. This is why dietary guidelines issued by the U.S. Department of Agriculture, the National Cancer Institute, and the American Heart Association recommend eating five or more daily servings of fruits and vegetables.

It is not known which of the many substances in fruits and vegetables might be responsible for the protection against disease, or why they are protective, but evidence indicates that "antioxidants" contribute substantially to the protection. Antioxidants, such as vitamins C, E and carotenes, can neutralize reactive oxygen species called "free radicals", which can damage body cells and initiate disease. Fruit and vegetables contain abundant amounts of natural antioxidants.

Recent research shows that smokers have lower blood

levels of antioxidants compared to non-smokers, even when dietary intakes are equal. Smoking produces an increased oxidative stress on the body, and the body's antioxidants are used up faster in smokers than in non-smokers. This effect has been officially recognized only for vitamin C, for which the RDA (Recommended Dietary Allowance) was increased to 100 mg per day for smokers compared 60 mg per day for non-smokers. Recent evidence suggests that recommended allowances for other protective nutrients also should be raised for smokers. Thus smokers, who have an increased risk of developing many degenerative diseases due to smoking itself, also have lower body levels of nutrients that are protective against disease.

In the following pages, Alistair Moodie provides important information that smokers should know about antioxidants and health and the changes that smokers can make in their diet to help protect their health if they continue to smoke. Besides quitting smoking, the most useful change that smokers can make is to increase their intake of fruits and vegetables. Supplementing the diet with antioxidants is a secondary choice because there are many antioxidants in plants which are not yet isolated and available in supplement form. Also, many components of fruits and vegetables may protect against disease through actions other than antioxidant protection.

The author summarizes a great deal of information related to smoking, vitamins and health in a unique and interesting way. More importantly, this book offers a practical understanding of the special nutritional perils that smokers face, and the steps they can take to reduce their risks of developing disease.

**Hans-Anton Lehr MD, PhD,
University of Washington Medical Center,
Seattle, Washington.**

Let's face it: SMOKING IS DANGEROUS TO YOUR HEALTH - and no one can pretend they haven't heard. However despite the well documented health risks about 25% of adults in the United States, 46 million people, continue to smoke.

Interestingly more than two thirds of smokers express a desire to quit at least once every year, but only one in 40 does so with lasting success. The failure of so many smokers to quit the habit is largely due to the addictive action of nicotine, one of the major constituents of cigarette smoke.

Although many smokers may feel socially excluded by the ever increasing number of smoke-free restaurants, airplanes, workplaces and public areas, biomedical science has not abandoned them. Researchers have been successful not only in establishing an irrefutable link between cigarette smoking and many health hazards, but have also made major progress in identifying the mechanisms by which cigarette smoking exerts its harmful action. Only when you have recognized your enemy and identified his weaponry, can you devise effective means of protection.

This is exactly what is going on in biomedical science. The identification of harmful free radicals in cigarette smoke and in the lungs and blood stream of smokers has been a major advancement and has helped our understanding of how cigarette smoke causes damage to lungs and blood vessels leading to canccr. Indeed, one single puff of a cigarette contains one hundred trillion (100,000,000,000,000) free radicals, most which are inhaled into the lungs and find there way into the blood stream.

Yet, our bodies are not without effective means of protection against these free radicals. Antioxidants constantly fight and neutralize free radicals which are both generated in our organism during the normal wear and tear of body functions, and are also inflicted upon us in the form of food, sun beams, automobile exhaust fumes and other environmental pollutants, and - last but not least - cigarette smoke. Unfortunately, cigarette smoking additionally reduces antioxidant blood and tissue levels substantially, leaving smokers more vulnerable to the harmful action of free radicals.

And this is where the SMOKERS GUIDE TO VITAMINS AND HEALTH comes in: the most powerful antioxidants which we can use to boost our antioxidant defense system are also easily available in dietary vitamins and minerals, and even in green tea. We just need to know about them. Science has provided us with valuable clues, linking diets low in antioxidants with disease and diets rich in antioxidants with health. These findings are particularly important for the smoker.

Alistair Moodie has undertaken a major project in sifting through the scientific literature for these clues and has presented them to the public in a clear and understandable manner. The time is right for this book. Antioxidant diets and dietary supplements are safe, cheap, and available, and their impact on human health is impressive.

May this book find its way into the hands and minds of all those who know about the health risk they face by cigarette smoking, who have been unsuccessful in forsaking the highly addictive habit, but who can now actively do something to reduce their risk.

Harinder S. Garewal MD, PhD,
Professor of Medicine,
Cancer Prevention & Control Program,
University of Arizona Health Sciences Center,
Tucson, Arizona.

A well-researched, easy to read, current manuscript addressing a rapidly evolving field. Smokers should discontinue smoking! Hardly anyone, smoker or non-smoker, will argue otherwise. Nevertheless, for many, this is easier said than done.

Nutritional factors have a role in disease occurrence and prevention! Another statement few will disagree with. Many studies have suggested that smokers not only often have poorer dietary habits, but also metabolize nutrients differently and require increased intakes of "good" nutrients to maintain blood and tissue levels comparable with non-smokers.

Moodie has succinctly put together the findings of numerous studies and has done an admirable job of presenting this information in a balanced manner. Stop smoking and pay attention to nutrition (whether you stop smoking or not) is sound advice for disease prevention and health promotion. That smoking tobacco affects nutritional needs, and how one handles nutrients, is the take home message for smokers who just can't quit. As in any endeavor of this nature, there will be controversies surrounding one specific recommendation or the other. Furthermore, the field continues to evolve as more is learned with each new completed study. In this environment of active, ongoing modulation of the state of knowledge, this book constitutes a valuable resource for smokers as they continue their attempts to stop smoking.

1

How Smokers Can Protect Their Health

After decades of health warnings from the Surgeon General and other health authorities few people would now deny that smoking carries health risks. However despite these risks over 46 million Americans, about one fourth of the adult population, choose to smoke.

If you are part of this much neglected and persecuted group, it is for you this book is written. Here you will find described the many steps you can take to reduce the risks of smoking and protect your health.

The book summarizes the results of more than 200 scientific studies on smoking, vitamins and health. A great number of these studies show a strong and consistent link between a high intake of antioxidant vitamins or fruits and vegetables rich in antioxidant vitamins and reduced risk of smoking related diseases. Also included are other simple changes you can make in the foods you eat which offer health protection for smokers.

Increasing your intake of fruit and vegetables, taking vitamin supplements or changing your food choices are all simple and inexpensive ways you can protect your health.

A Little History

Medical science has conquered the major infectious diseases smallpox, tuberculosis, typhoid, cholera by finding an antidote to the microbe or foreign invader responsible for the infection. We now have vaccines to prevent these diseases or treatments to clear them up quickly when they occur.

Unfortunately the ailments from which most people in the industrialized world now suffer are the degenerative diseases such as cancer, heart disease, arthritis and cataract. Unlike infectious diseases which can lay you low or kill you in a matter of weeks or even days, it takes years or in some cases decades for the degenerative diseases to get the better of you. The infectious diseases of old have now been conquered, but unfortunately for the degenerative diseases, modern medical science has no quick and easy answers.

It is now widely accepted that these degenerative diseases are the result not of a single foreign agent invading the body but come about when a number of factors overwhelm the body's defenses. As this is a book for smokers, let's take lung cancer as an example. Most people, including smokers, now accept that smoking is a cause of lung cancer. However not all smokers get lung cancer and on the other hand about 8% of people who have never smoked are struck down with this disease. Factors other than smoking must play a part. What you eat, atmospheric pollution, lack of exercise, lack of sleep, stress and probably several other factors all contribute to weaken our bodies defense system and increase vulnerability to this cancer and many other diseases.

The Importance of What You Eat

In the 1970s population surveys began to show a consistent link between a diet rich in fruit and vegetables and lowered rates of cancer and heart disease. Attention then turned to examining the results of these studies nutrient by nutrient to uncover the link with specific ailments.

Vitamin C, vitamin E and beta carotene, known as the antioxidants, soon took center stage as the evidence continued to build. The point has now been reached where several hundred scientific studies link a high intake of these antioxidant vitamins or foods rich in them with reduced risk of heart disease and cancer, especially lung cancer. There is little need to remind you here that as a smoker these are the ailments from which you are most at risk.

Smokers and Vitamins - The Bad News and The Good News

The bad news - Several large scale surveys have measured the antioxidant vitamin status of smokers compared to nonsmokers and consistently report the following:

1) smokers have lower intake of antioxidant vitamins
2) smokers use up antioxidant vitamins more rapidly
3) smokers have lower blood and tissue levels of these vitamins.

In other words smokers are nearly always deficient in the essential antioxidant vitamins which have shown a strong and consistent link with reduced risk of heart disease, lung cancer and a wide range of other ailments associated with smoking.

The good news - Fortunately increasing your intake and raising your blood and tissue levels of the antioxidant vitamins is not difficult. Broadly speaking you have three choices:

● Change your diet. Increasing the amount of fresh fruits and vegetables you eat will raise your intake of vitamin C and carotenes. This is the best way to get your daily needs of these two vitamins as scientists believe fruits and vegetables may contain other as yet undiscovered protective nutrients.

● Take vitamin supplements. If you are unable, or do not choose to eat the recommended quantities of fruits and vegetables to get sufficient vitamin C and carotenes then you have the option to take supplements.

As it is nearly impossible to get sufficient vitamin E from foods to reach the level at which protective effects have been found, taking supplements is the only way to go for this vitamin.

● Combine the two. Do your best to increase your intake of fresh fruits and vegetables and take vitamin supplements to ensure your intake of these nutrients reaches the level which gives optimum health and provides maximum protection from disease.

2

What are Antioxidant Vitamins and How Do They Work

Free Radicals and Antioxidants

Oxygen, the life sustaining gas in the air we breathe, is essential to our survival. Our bodies use oxygen to produce energy which enables us to power our muscles and do all the wonderful things we humans can do. This energy production process, which scientists call oxidation is very efficient, but like most things, comes at a price. During the process destructive by-products, known as free radicals are released into our bodies. These free radicals can damage virtually every cell in the body, by corroding the cell membrane, its outer protective skin, by altering the DNA code, the human blueprint or by killing cells outright.

Most people are familiar with everyday examples of the

oxidation process - the browning of an apple when cut, the rusting of metal and the way butter goes rancid. The majority of scientists now believe the chaos and destruction caused by free radicals plays a major role in development of degenerative diseases such as cancer, heart disease, arthritis and cataract. There is also strong evidence pointing to free radical damage as the major cause of the gradual deterioration we call aging.

Strong support for the free radical theory of aging emerged recently in an article in Science magazine, February 1994. Biologists at Southern Methodist University in Dallas, Texas published their report on a study of fruit flies. They discovered that flies geneticly engineered to resist free radical damage live up to one third longer than normal flies.

The Body's Answer to the Free Radical Problem

Fortunately the body has a natural defense system to combat damaging free radical attacks. Compounds known as antioxidants act like cops, hunting down free radicals and neutralizing them. Some of these protective antioxidants occur naturally in the body but several others can only be obtained from food. So far the most important antioxidants found in food are vitamin C, vitamin E and beta carotene.

In nature this internal battle between the bad guys, the free radicals, and the good guys, the antioxidants is more or less in balance. However in our modern industrialized world two factors have shifted this balance against us.

Firstly - free radical attacks have intensified. Industrial pollution, car exhaust fumes and other contaminants all increase our body's intake of free radicals from the environment. Unfortunately cigarette smoke also carries a heavy load of free radicals.

Secondly - our defense systems are weakened. The fast paced American lifestyle with long work hours and two income families means less time to buy and prepare fruits and vegetables, the food source of antioxidant vitamins.

Tipping the Scales in Your Favor

A high intake of fruits and vegetables has been shown to provide substantial protection from many of the degenerative diseases. The National Cancer Institute, the National Academy of Sciences, the American Health Foundation and the US Department of Agriculture have all issued dietary guidelines for Americans. These recommend we eat at least five, and preferably more servings of fruit and vegetables every day to help protect us from cancer and heart disease.

Unfortunately large scale federal surveys reveal that over 90% of Americans don't reach these dietary goals. If you are part of this 90% then you should do all you can to increase your intake of fruit and vegetables to the recommended levels. However if you find this difficult, and many people do, then taking vitamin supplements is the next best alternative and provides insurance against most deficiencies.

The RDAs - A Little History

You can't talk about vitamins and minerals for very long without coming across the Recommended Dietary Allowances or RDAs, so a few words of explanation are in order.

Nutrition research originally focused on vitamins and their role in combating the deficiency diseases, for example vitamin C to prevent scurvy, vitamin D to prevent rickets, and vitamin B1 to prevent beriberi. From these studies came the Recommended Dietary Allowances or RDAs originally formulated during World War 2 as the minimum nutrition levels necessary to prevent the deficiency diseases being found in military recruits. These are the RDAs you will find today on vitamin supplement labels and breakfast cereal packets.

However in the last decade or so, nutrition science and the study of vitamins has entered what many are calling the "second wave". This latest nutrition research focuses on optimal health and the avoidance of disease, especially the degenerative, diseases cancer, heart disease, cataract etc.

It is this "second wave" of nutrition research which has shown a strong and consistent link between the intake of antioxidant vitamins at doses much above the RDAs and the prevention of many diseases, offering us all the possibility of staying healthier and living longer.

The next four chapters will examine the latest scientific evidence on the individual antioxidant vitamins, the protection they offer and how smokers can benefit.

Full references for all studies quoted are given at the end of the book

3

Beta Carotene and Your Health

What Beta Carotene Can Do For You

Beta carotene has been receiving a lot of media coverage lately, hardly a day goes by without some newspaper, magazine or TV news spot telling the benefits of this "newly discovered" nutrient.

All this attention is well deserved as there is strong and consistent evidence linking a high intake of carotenes or foods rich in carotenes with greatly reduced risk of the following:

● Lung cancer
● Heart disease
● Cataract of the eye

There is also good evidence linking high blood beta carotene levels to reduced risk of cancer of the mouth and throat, lung and gynecological cancers.

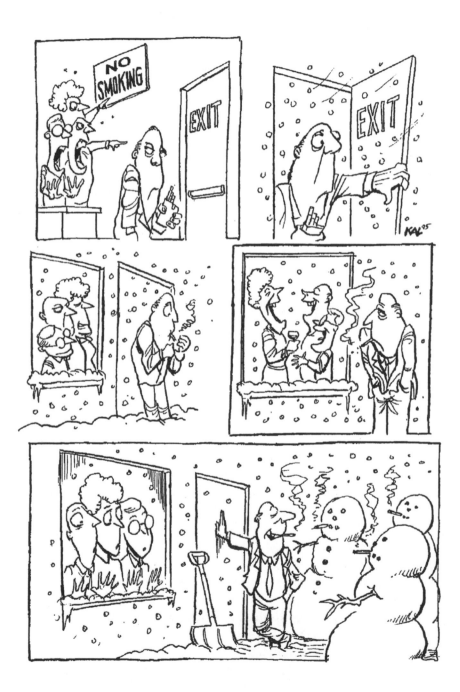

What Are Carotenes

Carotenes, sometimes called carotenoids, are a group of over 600 naturally occurring substances which give many fruits and vegetables their yellow or orange/red coloring.

Of the many carotenes found in food only a few are present in sufficient quantities to play a significant role in human nutrition. Beta carotene which accounts for about 25% of food carotenes plays a large role, but other carotenes such as lycopene, alpha carotene, beta cryptoxanthin, lutein and zeaxanthin are also believed to be important. These carotenes are present in various quantities in everyday foods, sweet potatoes and carrots are rich in beta carotene and tomatoes and watermelon are rich in lycopene.

There are carotenes in green vegetables but their distinctive colors are masked by the greens of chlorophyll, a major component of the energy production system of plants. However the distinctive carotene colors make their appearance in the fall when the chlorophyll disappears from the leaves on trees and the brilliant reds, oranges and yellows are exposed.

Although often called a vitamin, beta carotene is in fact a pro-vitamin. Scientists use the term pro-vitamin to describe any substance which the body can convert to a vitamin and in the case of beta carotene the body is able to convert it to vitamin A. Interest in beta carotene first came about as a result of its ability to convert to vitamin A, itself an essential nutrient, but it soon became clear that beta carotene was associated with powerful nutritional benefits of its own.

Beta carotene is the carotene which has received the most attention in the field of human nutrition. Part of the reason is it is the only carotene available on a commercial basis, having been used as a food colorant for many years - most margarines get their color from beta carotene.

How Beta Carotene Works

It appears that beta carotene protects cells in two ways. Firstly it is a fat soluble antioxidant which can neutralize free radicals and secondly, and probably more important, it is a most effective naturally occurring neutralizer of the singlet oxygen molecule. This molecule is not itself a free radical but its high energy level and reactive nature leads to the production of enormous numbers of destructive free radicals.

Specific features in the make up of beta carotene enable it to neutralize singlet oxygen molecules thus preventing the production of free radicals and yet remaining unchanged itself. Laboratory tests show that one molecule of beta carotene can neutralize up to 1000 singlet oxygen molecules.

How Beta Carotene Dosage is Measured

Beta carotene dosage is usually given in International Units, written in abbreviated form as "IU" and this is how you will find it listed on most supplement labels. An International Unit is simply a universally accepted measure of the amount of active ingredient. The most common supplement dosage of beta carotene is 25,000 IU but you can also find 10,000 IU and 50,000 IU doses.

The more correct way to measure beta carotene dosage is in milligrams abbreviated "mg" as this is the way all other carotenes are measured. You can convert beta carotene dosage from one to another using the following formula:

10,000 IU = 6 mg
1 mg = 1666 IU

Are You Getting Enough Beta Carotene.

The sad fact is that if you eat a typical American diet then you are probably not getting enough beta carotene and related carotenes.

Although the most plentiful carotene in human food, beta carotene is fairly new to the field of nutrition study and as yet there is no recommended level of intake. This led Paul Lachance, Professor of Food Science at Rutgers University down the investigative trail. He examined the diets recommended by the National Cancer Institute's Guide to Food Choices and the US Department of Agriculture's recommended dietary goals.

By calculating the amount of carotenes, as vitamin A, in each of the foods in these diets he was able to discover how much beta carotene equivalent would be consumed if these diets were followed. His calculations show they would provide a daily intake of about 10,000 IU (6 mg) of beta carotene or its equivalent.

So how much carotene does the average American consume? The US Department of Agricultures's 1985/86 Continuing Survey of Food Intakes of Individuals reveals that Americans are consuming only 2,500 IU (1.5 mg) of beta carotene or its equivalent per day. This is only one fourth of the level these ideal diets would provide. The situation for smokers is even worse.

Smoking and Beta Carotene

Since 1982 there have been five studies which have looked at the level of beta carotene in smokers blood and all found smokers had lower levels than nonsmokers.

One of these studies in 1988, by researchers at Harvard School of Public Health showed that blood levels of beta carotene were much lower in smokers than in nonsmokers despite the fact their diets were similar. Men who smoked a pack of cigarettes a day had a blood beta carotene level 28%

lower than nonsmokers, for women the figure was 21% lower.

Evidence linking the eating of foods containing carotenes with lower incidence of lung, digestive tract and other cancers has led the National Academy of Sciences to recommend all Americans increase their consumption of carotene rich foods.

Carotenes and Lung Cancer

According to the 1989 Surgeon General's report male smokers are 22 times more likely and female smokers 12 times more likely to get lung cancer than non-smokers.

● A study published in 1993 of data collected from residents of Hawaii looked at the protective effects of several carotenes. Researchers found that men with the highest intake of beta carotene equivalents had only half the risk of contracting lung cancer compared to men with lowest intake. For women, the highest intake of beta carotene equivalents cut the risk of lung cancer by 65% compared to those with the lowest intake.

● In 1991 Suzanne Gaby, Adjunct Professor of Nutrition at New York University, compiled a survey of 30 studies on beta carotene and the risk of lung cancer. Some of the studies measured the beta carotene consumed in daily food intake, while others measured the level of beta carotene in the blood. The results were published in the book "Vitamin Intake and Health", Marcel Dekker, 1991.

Of the 30 studies, 26 found that individuals with a high intake of foods rich in beta carotene or high blood levels of beta carotene gained a substantial degree of protection from lung cancer compared with those with lowest intake or blood levels. On average the risk of lung cancer was cut by 50%. Here are three examples of these studies:

● The Western Electric Study - Researchers followed the diets and eating habits of nearly 2,000 men employed by Western Electric Company in Chicago over a 19 year period. With the help of charts showing the nutrient content of various foods, daily intakes of carotene were calculated. The men were divided into four groups depending on their carotene intake. At the end of the study results showed that the group with the lowest intake of carotenes were seven times more likely to get lung cancer compared to the group with the highest intake.

● The Washington County Study - In 1974 blood samples from 25,000 residents of Washington County, Maryland were collected and preserved by freezing. Over the next 9 years all cases of lung cancer were recorded and the blood samples from these lung cancer patients unfrozen and tested for beta carotene level.

When scientists from Johns Hopkins School of Public Health in Baltimore studied the results, they found that individuals with low blood levels of beta carotene were twice as likely to get lung cancer compared with those who had the highest levels.

● The Basel, Switzerland Study - In 1973 a group of Swiss researchers measured the antioxidant blood levels of nearly 3000 male volunteers employed by local chemical companies. The men were then followed for 12 years and all cases of cancer recorded. When the results were analyzed they showed that individuals with the lowest blood carotene levels had over twice the risk of lung cancer compared to those with the highest levels.

Tobacco is a dirty weed: I like it.
It satisfies no normal need. I like it.
It makes you thin, it makes you lean,
It takes the hair right off your bean,
It's the worst darn stuff I've ever seen,
I like it.

Graham Hemminger,
Published in the "Penn State Froth" newspaper, 1915.

Researchers in this study ended their report by encouraging a higher intake of carotenes or supplements containing carotenes as a preventive measure against cancer. They also stressed that their data showed smokers had consistently lower carotene blood levels.

● The Finnish Study - A report published in Spring 1994 from a study in Finland made media headlines. Researchers followed Finnish males, 50 to 69 years of age, who had smoked more than 20 cigarettes a day for an average of 35 years. Their results suggested that taking beta carotene supplements increased the risk of lung cancer.

These results were baffling. Even the researchers who wrote the report were puzzled as the findings differed so markedly from the many other studies which showed positive benefits of a high carotene intake from food. Critics of the study point out that about 1 in 5 of the participants had been exposed to cancer hazards in their jobs as asbestos installers, miners and foundry workers and were therefore an unsuitable study group.

To add further confusion the researchers also discovered that in the group receiving no supplements, the higher the blood beta carotene level they had at the beginning of the survey, the lower their risk of lung cancer.

The authors of the report, writing in the New England Journal of Medicine, stated "we are aware of no other data at this time ... that suggest harmful effects of beta carotene, whereas there are data indicating benefit." They also added "in the light of all the data available, an adverse effect of beta carotene seems unlikely ... this finding may well be due to chance".

What do these results say about beta carotene and lung

cancer risk? There are two possibilities:-
1) Something else other than beta carotene was responsible for the reduction in lung cancer risk in all those other studies. Some other component of fruits and vegetables, the main source of beta carotene, provided the protection.
2) It may be that if you have been smoking for a long time, 35 years was the average in this study, it is too late for beta carotene to be of any benefit.

So what's the bottom line? This study raises a caution flag with regard to beta carotene supplements and lung cancer. However, what you can do is eat a diet rich in fruits and vegetables. This will provide you not only with beta carotene but all the other carotenes and all other components of fruits and vegetables which may be responsible for the protection from lung cancer.

Carotenes and Heart Disease

Most people when asked to name a health risk associated with smoking would say "lung cancer". However heart disease is really the number one enemy, as each year it kills many more smokers than lung cancer, although both take a heavy toll.

Smokers are approximately twice as likely to get heart disease as non smokers.

● On May 20th, 1993 the results of a Harvard School of Public Health study made the front page of the New York Times. The study which followed the dietary habits of 120,000 men and women strongly suggested that vitamin E supplements significantly reduce the risk of heart disease.

Not mentioned in the headlines was another set of results from the same study. These showed that for smokers there was a dramatic link between high carotene intake and reduced risk of heart disease. Smokers with the highest carotene intake, more than 14,388 IU per day, cut their risk of heart disease by 70% compared to those with the lowest intake who consumed less than 5030 IU per day.

● In November 1994, researchers at the School of Medicine at the University of North Carolina published the results of a study on carotenes and risk of heart disease. The blood carotene levels of 3,806 men with high cholesterol were measured at the start of the trial and all cases of coronary heart disease during the 13 year follow-up period were noted.

When the results were tabulated, smokers in the group who had high carotene blood levels were 22% less likely to suffer from heart disease than smokers with low carotene blood levels.

● Results from a recent European study confirm the connection between beta carotene and reduced risk of heart disease. Scientists compared 683 heart disease patients with a similar number of healthy individuals all taken from ten different European locations. Smokers with low tissue levels of beta carotene were over twice as likely to suffer from heart disease than smokers with high tissue levels.

Carotenes and Cataract

Cataract is the progressive clouding of the lens of the eye leading eventually to blindness. Exposure to ultraviolet light from the sun's rays is believed to be the major cause and not surprisingly, cataracts are more common in countries which have sunny climates.

In the US the great majority of cataracts are found in older Americans. As we age damaged tissue gradually builds up in the lens as a result of long term exposure to light. By age 70 approximately 18% of Americans have cataracts and by the time we reach 80 the figure has risen to 45%. Cataract extraction is the most frequent operation performed on elderly Americans, accounting for 1.2 million surgeries every year.

Paying for cataract extractions costs Medicare $3.3 billion every year and is the single most expensive item, accounting for approximately 12% of total budget.

● Smoking has also been linked to increased risk of cataract. Two recent major studies by researchers at Harvard Medical School's Channing Laboratory produced strong evidence that smoking more than doubles the risk of cataract. Dr Sheila West of the Dana Center for Preventive Opthalmolgy in Baltimore, writing in the Journal of the American Medical Association estimates that 20% of cataracts are the result of smoking.

● Researchers Paul Jacques and Leo Chylack at the US Department of Agriculture's Human Nutrition Research Center on Aging at Tufts University in Boston ran a study on vitamins and the risk of cataract. The diets and vitamin supplement intake of seventy-seven people with cataract were compared with a matched group showing no sign of cataract.

Blood samples were taken and analyzed for vitamin status. Results showed that individuals with lowest blood carotene levels had over 5 times the risk of cataract compared to those with the highest.

● In 1992 Paul Knekt, head of a group of researchers at the Social Insurance Institute in Helsinki, Finland ran a study on antioxidant vitamins and cataract risk. The results confirmed the findings of previous studies, the lower the blood level of beta carotene the greater the risk of cataract.

Strong evidence suggests a high intake of beta carotene, vitamin C and vitamin E taken together produce the greatest cataract risk reduction.

Mouth and Throat Cancers

Researcher Harinder Garewal at the University of Arizona Medical Center has shown in several studies that beta carotene can safely prevent or reverse oral leukoplakia, a precancerous lesion which can lead to oral cancer. This protective effect has been confirmed by several other researchers in the field. Tobacco, either smoked or chewed, is responsible for over 75% of oral cavity cancers.

Garewal has also found that patients given beta carotene show a significant increase in several immune system responses.

Breast and Gynecological Cancers

Researchers Suzanne Gaby and Vishna Singh reviewed 14 studies on the link between beta carotene intake or beta carotene blood level and the risk of gynecological cancers.

Four out of six studies on breast cancer showed reduced risk with a high intake or a high blood level of beta carotene.

Seven out of eight studies on cervical and endometrial cancers showed reduced risk with a high intake or a high blood level of beta carotene.

How to Get Your Carotenes - Foods or Supplements

The evidence linking a high carotene blood level, a high

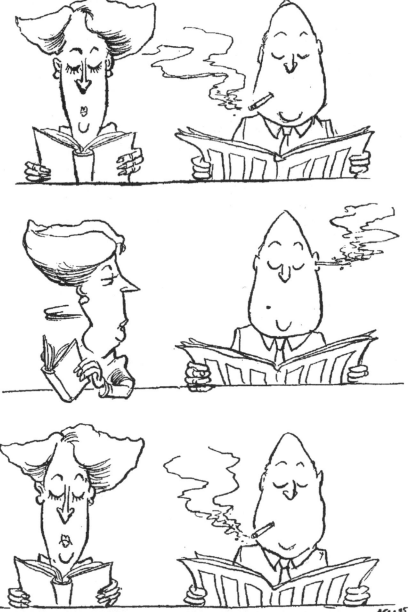

intake of carotenes or foods rich in carotenes to greatly reduced risk of cancer, especially lung cancer, is strong and consistent. For heart disease there is good evidence of strong protection, especially for smokers. As these diseases are the two major health hazards for smokers, you should make every effort to raise your intake, the higher the better. Eat five and preferably more servings of carotene rich fresh fruit and vegetables every day, the dark green and yellow vegetables are especially important for smokers.

A quick reference table giving the best sources for the five major carotenes is shown below and a detailed table of the beta carotene content of various foods is given at the end of the chapter.

Carotene Rich Foods

For each carotene listed, the first food is the richest source, the further along each list you go the less rich the source.

Alpha carotene: pumpkin, carrots (raw, cooked, canned, or frozen).

Beta carotene: sweet potatoes, carrots (raw, cooked, canned, frozen), spinach, collard greens, apricots, canned pumpkin, cantaloupe.

Beta cryptoxanthin: papaya, oranges, tangerines.

Lutein and Zeaxanthin: kale, collard greens, spinach, swiss chard, mustard greens, red pepper, okra, romaine lettuce.

Lycopene: tomato juice, guava, watermelon, pink grapefruit, tomatoes.

All comparisons on a weight for weight basis.

Beta Carotene

As shown earlier, following the health protecting diets recommended by the US Department of Agriculture and the National Cancer Institute would provide you with about 10,000 IU of beta carotene or its equivalent per day. But the sad fact is most people get only about 2,500 IU per day and for smokers the figure is even lower.

Eating carotene rich foods is the best answer, but if you have difficulty getting your five servings of carotene rich foods every day, then it makes sense to take a beta carotene supplement. The suggested dose is 10,000 IU. Supplements of 10,000 IU are available from many sources and many multivitamin tablets contain 10,000 IU.

How Safe is Beta Carotene

A rare inherited disease called erythropoietic protoporphyria causes super sensitivity to sunlight and sufferers from the disease are forced to keep all skin surfaces covered or stay indoors protected from sunlight. If they are exposed to the sun their skin turns red and burns in a matter of minutes.

An alert scientist, Dr Mathews-Roth, noting that beta carotene protected plants from sun damage, suggested that beta carotene supplements might help improve this condition. Her hunch turned out to be correct, and beta carotene has been used to treat inherited sun sensitivity diseases for 15 years. Many patients have taken doses of 300,000 IU every day for years with no adverse effects other than yellowing of the skin.

The Food and Drug Administration has approved beta carotene as a color additive for use in foods and the safety of beta carotene supplements at doses of 25,000 to 80,000 IU per day (15-50mg/day) has been demonstrated in numerous studies.

At daily doses of 25,000 IU and above beta carotene may cause a yellowing of the skin. This condition is harmless and disappears when the dosage is reduced.

Beta Carotene and Other Antioxidants

Beta carotene has been shown to boost the action of vitamin C and vitamin E. Using all three together appears to give an effect greater than the sum of their individual effects.

Odds and Ends

● Regular drinkers of alcohol have low blood levels of beta carotene with still lower levels seen in drinkers who smoke.
● A study conducted by researchers from the National Cancer Institute discovered that beta carotene is much more easily absorbed from supplements than from food.

Summary

For the smoker, at greatly increased risk from lung cancer, heart disease and cataract of the eye, a high intake of carotenes offers the potential of strong protective benefits. If your intake of carotene rich foods is low then taking a 10,000 IU (6 mg) beta carotene supplement is the next best alternative. The cost is low, the benefits great and the safety factor very high.

Beta Carotene Content of Common Foods

(all nutrient levels are approximate and will vary)

FOOD	SERVING SIZE	IU	mg
FRUITS			
Apricots, fresh	2	4,100	2.5
Apricots, dried	10 halves	10,300	6.2
Cantaloupe	1/2	8,000	4.8
Grapefruit, pink or red	1/2	2,600	1.6
Mango	1/2	2,300	1.4
Watermelon	1 slice	1,800	1.1
VEGETABLES, cooked unless otherwise stated			
Bell peppers, raw	1/2 cup	1,800	1.1
Beet greens	1/2 cup	3,000	1.8
Broccoli	1/2 cup	1,600	1.0
Carrot, raw	1 medium	9,500	5.7
Chicory, raw	1 cup	10,300	6.2
Collard greens	1/2 cup	5,600	3.4
Dandelion greens	1/2 cup	2,300	1.4
Kale	1/2 cup	5,000	3.0
Mustard greens	1/2 cup	3,100	1.9
Pumpkin	1/2 cup	6,100	3.7
Romaine lettuce, raw	1 cup	1,800	1.1

Beta carotene content of common foods, cont'd

FOOD	SERVING SIZE	IU	mg
Spaghetti squash	1/2 cup	3,100	1.9
Spinach	1/2 cup	8,100	4.9
Spinach, raw	1 cup	3,800	2.3
Sweet potato	1 medium	16,000	10.0
Swiss chard	1/2 cup	5,300	3.2
Turnip greens	1/2 cup	6,500	3.9
Winter squash	1/2 cup	4,800	2.9
JUICES AND SOUPS			
Carrot juice	1 cup	40,000	24.2
Gazpacho	1 cup	19,600	11.7
Manhattan clam chowder	1 cup	3,100	1.9
Split pea soup	1 cup	2,300	1.4
Tomato juice	1 cup	3,600	2.2
Vegetable soup	1 cup	3,100	1.9
Vegetable and beef stew	1 cup	2,800	1.7

Sources:
Carotenoid content of fruits and vegetables: an evaluation of analytic data. Journal of the American Dietetic Association 93:3, 284-296, 1993.

Carotenoid analyses of selected raw and cooked foods associated with lower risk of cancer. Journal of the National Cancer Institute 82:282-285, 1990.

Sultan Murad IV of Turkey is typical of the early Eastern antismoking crusaders. Determined to enforce the royal no-smoking edict, Murad reportedly prowled the streets of seventeenth-century Istanbul incognito, accosting suspected tobacco sellers, begging them to sell him a small quantity, offering them payment far in excess of the going rate and swearing eternal secrecy. Then if the merchant's greed overcame his caution and he produced the forbidden substance, Murad would personally behead him on the spot, leaving the body in the street as a grisly warning. But despite Murad's efforts, smoking continued - prospered actually - in Turkey.

Poetic justice was served almost three centuries later, when Turkish tobacco cigarettes called "Murads" became one of America's most popular brands.

Reprinted with permission of "American Heritage" magazine.

4

Vitamin E and Smoker's Health

What Vitamin E Can Do For You

Results from many scientific studies show a strong and consistent link between a high intake of vitamin E and reduced risk of:
● Heart disease
● Lung disease (emphysema and bronchitis)
● Mouth, throat and esophageal cancer
● Cataract

What is Vitamin E

Vitamin E is the body's major fat soluble antioxidant and is an essential nutrient. As the body cannot manufacture its own supply, it must be provided by foods or supplements.

To the scientist the name vitamin E refers to a family of

compounds called tocopherols, which all have similar properties. The most important member of this family is d-alpha-tocopherol and you will sometimes find this name used for vitamin E. Don't be too concerned about these different names, for our purposes vitamin E is just vitamin E.

How Vitamin E Works

Vitamin E performs several different functions:
● It reduces blood platelet stickyness thought to be the primary cause of artery clogging which can result in heart attack and stroke.
● As the body's major fat soluble antioxidant, it protects critical cellular structures from free radical damage.
● It blocks the production of nitrosamines which are formed in the body, in the foods we eat, and in cigarette smoke. Nitrosamines are known cancer causing chemicals.

How Vitamin E Dosage is Measured

Vitamin E is measured in "International Units", usually abbreviated to "IU". International units are a universal standard of measure of the amount of active ingredient. Occasionally you will find vitamin E dosage measured in milligrams, abbreviated "mg". To convert one to the other use the formula:

$$1.49 \text{ IU} = 1 \text{ mg (d-alpha tocopherol)}$$

Vitamin E supplements are usually sold in softgel capsule form and in dosages of 100 IU, 200 IU, 400 IU and 1000 IU.

Are You Getting Enough Vitamin E

In 1990 a team of researchers from the National Cancer Institute and the University of California at Berkeley estimated the vitamin E intake of Americans. They used data on daily food consumption for 11,658 adults collected by the National Center for Health Statistics, a division of the Department of Health and Human Services. Results showed that 69% of men and 80% of women were getting less than their respective Recommended Dietary Allowance (RDA). The RDA for men is 15 IU and for women 12 IU.

Smoking and Vitamin E

Cigarette smokers have been found to have lower levels of vitamin E in the protective fluid film which coats the inner surface of the lungs. Many scientists believe this vitamin E protects the lungs from damage by free radicals found in cigarette smoke. Free radical induced lung damage can lead to emphysema and bronchitis. In a study detailed below smokers were found to have less than one sixth the amount of vitamin E in the lungs compared to non smokers.

● Researchers in Japan have found that lung cancer patients have lower blood levels of vitamin E compared to healthy individuals.

● A survey covering three towns in England measured the antioxidant nutrient intake of 2,340 male and female smokers, nonsmokers and past smokers. Results showed vitamin E intake was lowest in current smokers and highest in nonsmokers.

Vitamin E and Protection from Heart Disease

Smokers are twice as likely to suffer a heart attack as non smokers and heart disease is the number one killer of smokers. Every year about 200,000 Americans die of smoking related heart disease and many more are disabled.

We have all at some time suffered from cuts on the surface of the skin and seen the bleeding stop in a matter of minutes. The body's natural defense system comes to the rescue. Small particles in the bloodstream called platelets stick to the injury site and clump together. This vital function, known as aggregation or blood clotting, plugs the damaged area and prevents us from bleeding to death.

Unfortunately there is a downside to this wonderful process. Oxidation of fats in the bloodstream can cause platelets to become overactive, aggregating or clotting too easily. The platelets form clumps which stick to the inside of artery walls, the pipework which carries oxygen rich blood from the heart to all areas of the body. This process can lead to clogging of the arteries which eventually results in heart attack or stroke. Several studies show vitamin E can suppress overactive platelets and reduce platelet stickyness.

● In May 1993 two studies by researchers at Harvard University Medical School reported near identical results.

The first followed the food and vitamin supplement intake of more than 87,000 healthy female nurses, from 1980 to 1992. The results showed that nurses taking a daily supplement of at least 100 IU of vitamin E were 34% less likely to have a heart attack.

The second study followed nearly 40,000 male dentists, pharmacists and other health professionals and similar results were found. Men taking a daily supplement of at least 100 IU of vitamin E were 37% less likely to suffer a heart attack.

Both studies revealed that vitamin E from food gave no measurable protection, probably because few of those followed were getting more than 8 IU (eight) of vitamin E from their diets.

● In 1987 a group of Swiss researchers lead by Fred Gey published the results of a survey of studies from several countries which looked at vitamin blood levels and the risk of heart disease. His team found that people living in countries such as Italy, Switzerland and Northern Ireland where blood levels of vitamin E were high, had a low to medium rate of heart disease. By contrast, in Finland and Scotland where blood levels of vitamin E were found to be lower, the rate of heart disease was high.

● Anthony Verlangieri, a researcher at the University of Mississippi examined the link between vitamin E and clogging of the arteries. His team fed a group of monkeys a high cholesterol diet designed to produce clogging of the arteries. The monkeys were divided into two groups, half were given a vitamin E supplement and half a dummy pill.

Results showed that the animals receiving the vitamin E supplement had reduced artery blockage compared to the non-supplemented animals.

Even more interesting was the discovery that when they changed the non-supplemented group over to vitamin E some of the artery blockage could actually be reversed.

Vitamin E and Protection for the Lungs

A substance called alveolar fluid coats the inner surface of the lungs. It contains vitamin E and scientists believe this vitamin E, acting as an antioxidant, helps protect the lungs from damage by free radicals and other pollutants found in

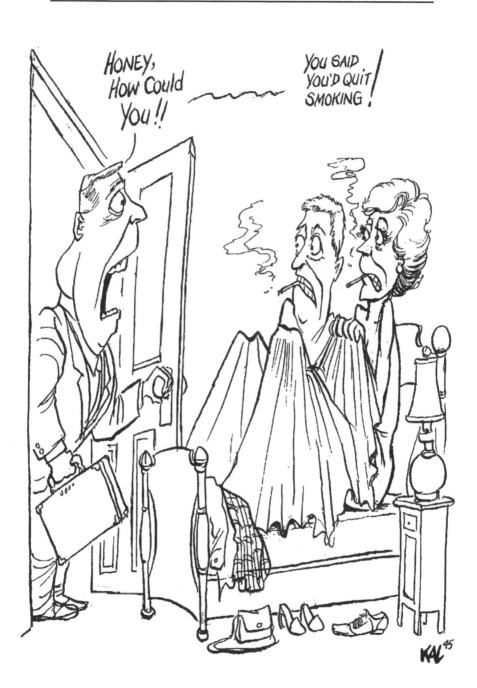

cigarette smoke. This free radical damage is thought to lead to emphysema and bronchitis.

● Eric Pacht and his co-workers in the Department of Medicine at Ohio State University ran a study to measure the vitamin E content of this lung fluid in both smokers and non-smokers. Their results showed that smokers had less than one sixth of the vitamin E compared to non-smokers.

● In 1974 blood samples from 25,000 Maryland residents were collected and preserved by freezing. Over the next 9 years all cases of lung cancer were recorded and the blood samples from these lung cancer patients unfrozen and tested for vitamin E level.

When scientists from Johns Hopkins School of Public Health in Baltimore sat down to study the results, they found that individuals with the lowest blood levels of vitamin E were nearly two and one half times more likely to get lung cancer compared with those who had the highest levels.

Mouth and Throat Cancer

In 1992 researchers at the National Cancer Institute published the results of a study into vitamin supplement use and the risk of mouth and throat cancer. The study followed individuals from four separate areas of the United States and found that for smokers, taking any vitamin E supplement cut the risk of mouth and throat cancer by 50%.

Vitamin E and Cataract

Details on smoking and the risk of cataract were given in the Beta Carotene chapter, but it bears repeating here that the evidence points to smokers having twice the risk of cataract compared to non smokers.

The two studies referred to in the cataract section of the beta carotene chapter also produced results for vitamin E.

The first by Paul Jacques and Leo Chylack at the US Department of Agriculture's Human Nutrition Research Center on Aging in Boston showed that individuals with a high intake of vitamin E had only half the risk of cataract compared to those with low intake.

The second study by Paul Knekt and his co-workers at the Social Insurance Institute in Helsinki, Finland showed a near doubling of cataract risk for individuals with a low intake of vitamin E compared to those with a high intake.

Results from one study show that people with a high intake of vitamins C and E and beta carotene had 80% less chance of developing cataract than those with a low intake.

Gastrointestinal Cancers

A 1993 study followed 35,000 Iowa women aged 55 to 69 to find out whether high intakes of antioxidant nutrients protected against colon cancer. At the end of the five year study period results showed that women with the highest intake of vitamin E were 68% less likely to get colon cancer than women with the lowest intake.

Immunity and Infection

Researchers at the US Department of Agriculture's Human Nutrition Research Center on Aging studied a group of healthy adults aged 60 years and over. They were given a daily supplement of 800 IU of vitamin E for one month. Results showed a boosting of their immune system.

How Much Vitamin E Do You Need

In the September 94 issue of "Health" magazine, Dr Gladys Block, Epidemiologist at University of California and Jeffrey Blumberg, Chief of the Antioxidant Research Laboratory at Tufts University, Boston, both stated they took a daily supplement of 400 IU of vitamin E.

The daily vitamin E supplement dosage of these two leading researchers, both nonsmokers, is in line with the dosage levels in the two major studies discussed in this chapter:
● Harvard Medical School studies - at least 100 IU per day required to show reduced risk of heart disease.
● The Basel study - suggest a prudent minimum daily intake of 60 - 100 IU

Remembering also the increased health risks run by smokers the suggested dose for maximum health protection is 100 - 400 IU per day.

Safety of Vitamin E

Vitamin E supplements are extremely safe. The strongest evidence was given in a series of strictly controlled studies where daily intakes of 600 - 3200 IU per day for 3 weeks to 6 months found very few side effects and none of which appeared consistently. Thousands of Americans have taken 400 IU or more of vitamin E for long periods with no side effects.

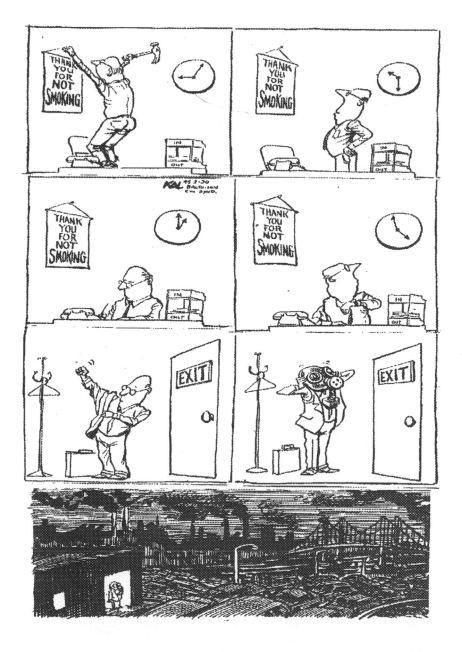

Who Shouldn't Take Vitamin E

People on anticoagulant therapy or taking vitamin K should not take vitamin E as this may interfere with their therapy. CONSULT YOUR PHYSICIAN.

Sources of Vitamin E

The richest sources are wheat germ oil, vegetable oils, egg yolk, nuts (especially sunflower seeds and almonds), green plants, milk fat and liver. Foods of animal origin are generally low in vitamin E.

It is however virtually impossible to get 100 IU or more from diet alone. To get 400 IU of vitamin E, considered an optimal dose by many experts, you would have to consume several cups of sunflower oil or its equivalent every day. Furthermore the oils and fats are undesirable sources of vitamin E as they are risk factors for heart disease and several cancers.

Odds and Ends

● Vitamin E has the reputation as an enhancer of sexual potency. The name tocopherol was first used by one of the discoverors of vitamin E. It comes from two Greek words, "tokos" meaning childbirth and the verb "phero" meaning to bring forth. Vitamin E was so named because it prevented reabsorbtion of the fetus in animals fed a rancid fat diet. Hence the name "bringer forth of childbirth" and the aphrodisiac and sexual potency myth followed.
● A large percentage of the vitamin E content of foods is destroyed by refining, processing and storing. Processing wheat into white flour destroys 92% of the vitamin E content,

thus wholegrain breads and cereals are better, plus the added bonus of the bran fiber content.

The bottom line

Many studies link a high intake of vitamin E, 100 IU per day or more, with reduced the risk of heart disease.

● It is nearly impossible to get 100 IU of vitamin E from food without consuming large quantities of polyunsaturated oils which add a considerable amount of fat to the diet.
● Considering the increased health risks to smokers, a daily supplement of 100 - 400 IU of vitamin E appears to offer the best health protection.

5

How Vitamin C Can Protect Your Health

Strong evidence from a wide range of scientific studies links a high intake of vitamin C or foods rich in vitamin C to reduced risk of the following:
- Lung and stomach cancer
- Heart disease and stroke
- Mouth and throat cancer
- Cataract
- Periodontal disease

Smokers are at greatly increased risk from all of the above and are routinely shown to be low in vitamin C.

Smokers Are Deficient in Vitamin C

Several food consumption surveys show that smokers get only slightly less vitamin C in their diet compared to nonsmokers. However when blood levels of vitamin C are examined, smokers are found to have much reduced levels. African-American smokers show particularly low vitamin C blood levels.

The reasons behind these reduced blood levels are not completely clear, but scientists believe that smokers use up and excrete vitamin C more quickly and there is good evidence absorption of vitamin C is poorer in smokers.

As early as 1968 a small study by Canadian researcher Omer Pelletier had shown that smokers had reduced blood vitamin C levels. Later in 1977 this same researcher ran a more comprehensive trial which looked at the blood vitamin C level of smokers and nonsmokers in various regions of Canada. He found that in comparison to nonsmokers, blood vitamin C levels were reduced by about 25% for smokers of less than 20 cigarettes a day and by about 40% for smokers of more than 20 cigarettes a day.

That smokers have low blood vitamin C levels was confirmed in a more recent study in 1989 by researchers at the Medical College of Wisconsin. After analyzing the blood samples from over 11,000 individuals their results showed smoking 20 cigarettes a day reduced blood vitamin C level by about 30% compared to nonsmokers.

Biological Sciences researcher Dr Akira Murata reviewed the results of 18 studies from 1963 through 1989 which looked at the smokers blood vitamin C levels. The results from every single study showed smokers had vitamin C blood levels lower than nonsmokers.

On average, smoking a pack or more a day reduces the level of vitamin C in the blood by up to 35% compared to nonsmokers. The greater the consumption of cigarettes the lower the blood level of vitamin C.

Every 10 years the US Federal Government conducts the National Health and Nutrition Examination Survey which is used to monitor the health and nutrition status of Americans. Data from the 1976-1980 survey showed that about 50% of smokers had vitamin C blood serum levels below normal.

Smokers also have another problem - lower levels of vitamin C in leukocytes, the white blood cells that destroy foreign bacteria and viruses which invade the body, including those associated with AIDS. A lower level of vitamin C in leukocytes is linked with reduced ability to protect cells and tissues from free radical damage.

● A study by scientists at Stanford University Center for Research in Disease Prevention found that people regularly exposed to second-hand smoke had lower blood levels of vitamin C compared to non-exposed nonsmokers. This is good reason for the family members of smokers to pay attention to their vitamin C intake.

What Is Vitamin C and How Does It Work

Vitamin C, also called ascorbic acid, is a nutrient essential for the proper functioning of the body. It is necessary for the production of collagen, the most common protein in the body and an essential building block for skin, cartilage, tendons, ligaments, bones, teeth and blood vessels. Unlike most animals humans cannot make vitamin C, they must get their daily needs from foods or supplements.

Vitamin C is water soluble and performs its powerful antioxidant function hunting down and destroying free radicals in water-based body fluids and tissue where the fat soluble vitamin E and beta carotene are less effective.

A cigarette is the perfect type of perfect pleasure. It is exquisite, and leaves one unsatisfied. What more can one want ?

Oscar Wilde,
"The Picture of Dorian Gray"

How Vitamin C Dosage Is Measured

Vitamin C dosage is measured in milligrams, abbreviated "mg", one thousand milligrams being equal to one gram. One gram is approximately equal to one twenty-eighth of an ounce.

Common vitamin C supplement doses are 250mg, 500mg and 1000mg.

Vitamin C and Protection from Heart Disease

Swiss researcher Fred Gey analyzed blood samples from groups of about 100 healthy middle aged men in Italy, Switzerland, Northern Ireland, Scotland and Finland. He measured the level of vitamin C in these blood samples and compared them with the death rate from heart disease in each country.

The results strongly suggest that the death rate from heart disease is lower in countries where blood levels of vitamin C are higher. The report ends by stating that normal healthy nonsmoking adults need at least 100 mg a day of vitamin C for maximum health protection.

● Hans-Anton Lehr and his research team at the University of Munich, in Germany recently reported their findings on vitamin C and cigarette smoke.

In a series of experiments on hamsters Dr Lehr showed that cigarette smoke causes leukocytes and platelets to aggregate and stick to the walls of arteries and veins. This process is believed to lead to both heart disease and the lung diseases emphysema and bronchitis.

In their most recent experiment these researchers showed that giving the hamsters vitamin C almost completely prevented leukocyte and platelet aggregation and adhesion.

The team ended its report by stating the levels of vitamin C which appeared to give protection for heart and lung diseases can easily be achieved in humans by dietary means or by taking supplements.

Vitamin C and Cancer Prevention

In 1991 National Cancer Institute researcher Gladys Block PhD reviewed 46 scientific studies on cancer and vitamin C intake. Almost all of the studies found a protective effect, with higher intakes halving the risk of cancer compared to lower intakes.

Her review covered an additional 30 studies which looked at the effect of eating fruits rich in vitamin C. Again almost all studies showed a protective effect, a high intake cutting the risk of cancer in half compared to low intake. Details of the results for the more common cancers are given below.

Lung cancer

Eleven studies looked at the link between lung cancer and vitamin C, five found a significant level of risk reduction with high intake, four showed a small protective effect and two showed no effect. Two studies which looked at fruit intake also found a protective effect against lung cancer.

Mouth and throat cancer

Smoking increases the risk of mouth and throat cancers.

There is strong evidence that vitamin C protects against mouth and throat cancer. Seven out of eight large well organized studies found that a high intake of vitamin C was linked to a lower risk of these cancers with several showing a halving of the risk with high intake compared to low intake. Eating foods rich in vitamin C also showed protective effects.

Stomach cancer

Eight studies looked at vitamin C intake and stomach cancer and all showed significant protection with a higher intake. A further eight studies examined the link between fruit intake and stomach cancer, and seven found a substantial risk reduction with higher intake.

Cancers of the colon and rectum

Six out of seven studies found reduced risk of rectal cancer with higher intake of vitamin C or foods rich in vitamin C.

For colon cancer six of eight studies found reduced risk with higher intake of vitamin C. One study found a 45% risk reduction when comparing high intake to low intake. A high intake of fruit was also found to be protective.

Cervical cancer

Several studies have found that a high intake of vitamin C or high blood levels of vitamin C were associated with a lower risk of cervical cancer and cervical dysplasia, a condition which can lead to cervical cancer.

A survey of dietary records revealed that women with vitamin C intake below 88mg per day had four times the risk of cervical dysplasia or cervical cancer compared to those with higher intake.

Pancreatic cancer

Several studies show a link between smoking and cancer of the pancreas, the fifth most common cause of cancer death in the United States. Unfortunately medical science has little to offer as treatment for this cancer and the outlook for sufferers is extremely poor. As a result preventive measures are of great importance.

Of the five studies on pancreatic cancer reviewed, all five found a significant protective effect from fruit. The one study which assessed vitamin C intake found that those consuming less than 70mg per day had two and a half times greater risk than those consuming 160mg per day or more.

Breast cancer

In 1990 the Journal of the National Cancer Institute published the results of a review of 12 studies on breast cancer and food intake. The results showed a consistent link between high intake of vitamin C and reduced risk of breast cancer. The authors of the review found that the degree of risk reduction associated with a high intake of vitamin C was at least equal to the risk reduction linked to a low fat diet.

Vitamin C and Cataract

As detailed in previous chapters, the best scientific estimates suggest that smoking doubles the risk of cataract and experts believe 20% of all cataracts are caused by smoking.

A 1991 study by James Robertson and his research team in the Medical School at the University of Western Ontario set out to examine the link between cataract and vitamin supplements. Two hundred and fifty patients with cataract, aged 55 and over were compared with a similar number who were cataract free. Results showed that individuals taking a vitamin C supplement of 300-600 mg per day cut their risk of cataract by 70%.

The study by Jacques and Chylack from Tufts University detailed in the chapter on beta carotene also looked at vitamin C and cataract. Results confirmed that both a high intake or high blood level of vitamin C were associated with a reduced risk of cataract.

Vitamin C, Sperm Count and Fertility

Cigarette smoking is associated with reduced sperm count and increased sperm abnormalities.

Studies have also revealed that normal semen has a high concentration of vitamin C, about eight times that of blood and as discussed earlier, smoking is also associated with lowered blood levels of vitamin C.

These facts led obstetrics and gynecology researchers at the University of Texas Medical Center to test whether vitamin C supplements could improve the sperm quality of smokers.

Seventy-five men aged 20-35 years, who all smoked at least a pack a day were divided into 3 groups. The first was given a dummy pill, the second 200mg/day of vitamin C and the third 1000mg/day of vitamin C. After four weeks the dummy pill group showed no improvement. Both vitamin C groups showed improved sperm quality with greater improvement in the group receiving the higher dose.

Results of a study by scientists at the University of California and the US dept of Agriculture's Western Human Nutrition Research Center showed similar results. Vitamin C protects human sperm from damage which could affect sperm quality and increase the risk of birth defects, particularly in those with low vitamin C such as smokers.

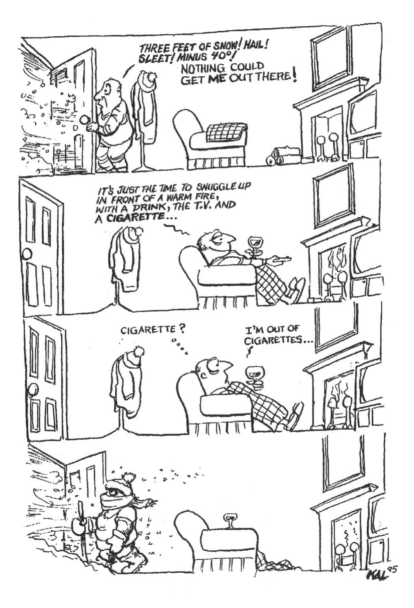

Vitamin C and Toxic Metals

Cigarette smoke contains high levels of toxic metals including lead. Vitamin C has been shown to bind with these toxic metals and aid in their elimination from the body, a process known as chelation.

Vitamin C and Periodontal Disease (gum disease)

According to a 1986 report by the US Department of Health and Human Services approximately 85% of adults have some periodontal disease. Experts are convinced that smoking increases the risk.

Bleeding gums and loosened teeth are two of the main symptoms of periodontal disease, and they are also the main symptoms of scurvy, the vitamin C deficiency disease. These two facts lead researchers to wonder if vitamin C could help prevent periodontal disease. The results of several studies do indeed show a link between increased intake or increased blood levels of vitamin C and improved gum health. However, an intake well above the Recommended Dietary Allowance was required to show protective benefits.

Vitamin C and the Immune System

There is some evidence that high doses of vitamin C stimulate the body's immune system which fights off foreign invaders such as bacteria and toxic particles.

How Much Vitamin C Do You Need

The US Food and Drug Administration recommends smokers get at least 100 mg of vitamin C per day, 66% above the recommended level for non smokers. Canada, New Zealand and France also recommend higher intake for smokers.

Several well respected researchers believe these levels may be too low and suggest an intake ranging from 140-210mg per day for smokers. Bear in mind that these recommendations are all based on the avoidance of scurvy, the vitamin C deficiency disease.

If optimum health and the prevention of disease is the desired result, then a vitamin C intake which produces tissue saturation is probably a good target to aim for. Tissue saturation is reached when additional amounts of vitamin C will not raise the amount stored in the body. Canadian researcher Omer Pelletier found that smokers required about 700 mg of vitamin C per day to reach saturation.

When all the evidence showing the strong and consistant link between a high intake of vitamin C or foods rich in vitamin C and reduced risk of smoking related ailments is considered, an intake of 500-1000 mg per day would appear to be an optimum level for smokers.

How to Get Your Vitamin C

As with beta carotene the ideal way to get your vitamin C is from foods as scientists believe that fruits and vegetables rich in vitamin C may contain other antioxidant nutrients which give protection from disease. However getting your intake up to 1000mg per day means you would have to drink 15 glasses of orange juice or the equivalent. For most people this is not a practical option.

The best solution is to eat as many fruits and vegetables as you can, and take a vitamin C supplement. If your vitamin C intake from fruits and vegetables is high then take a 500mg supplement, if your intake from fruits and vegetables is low, take a 1000mg supplement.

Charts showing the vitamin C content of fruits and vegetables are shown on the following pages.

Safety of Vitamin C

Vitamin C is very safe, the only consistent side effect is diarrhea at high doses, several thousand milligrams or more. This effect disappears when dosage is reduced.

One of the most persistent rumors about vitamin C is that large doses can produce kidney stones. Numerous scientific studies have failed to find any connection between a high intake of vitamin C and increased kidney stone formation. However, high doses of vitamin C are not recommended for kidney disease sufferers.

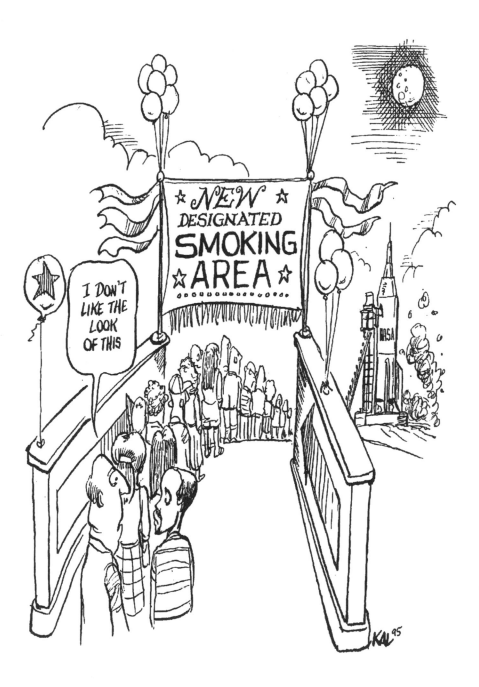

Vitamin C Content of Common Foods

All nutrient levels are approximate and will vary

Food	Serving Size	Vitamin C (mg)
FRESH FRUITS		
Apple, with skin	1 medium (3 per#)	8
Apricots	3 medium (12 per #)	11
Avocado	1 medium	16
Banana	1 medium (8-3/4" long)	10
Blackberries	1/2 cup	15
Blueberries	1/2 cup	9
Raspberries	1/2 cup	15
Strawberries	1/2 cup	42
Cherries, sweet	10 cherries	5
Grapefruit	1/2	41
Orange	1 medium (2-3/4" diam)	70
Pumello	1/2 cup of sections	58
Tangerine	1 medium (2-2/8" diam)	26
Grapes	10 grapes	5
Guava	1 medium	165
Kiwifruit	1 medium	74
Mango	1/2	29
Melon, cantaloupe	1/2 medium (5" diam)	112
Melon, casaba	1/10 (7-3/4" x 2")	26
Melon, honeydew	1/10 (7" x 2")	32
Melon, watermelon	1 slice (10" x 1")	46

Vitamin C content of common foods cont'd

Nectarene	1 medium (2-1/2" diam)	7
Papaya	1/2 medium (3-1/2" diam)	94
Peach	1 medium (4 per #)	6
Pear	1 medium (2-1/2 per #)	7
Pineapple	1 slice (3-1/2" diam x 3/4")	13
Plum	1 medium (2-1/8" diam)	6

JUICES

Cranberry juice cocktail	6 fl oz	80
Grapefruit, canned, unsweetened	6 fl oz	54
Orange, canned	6 fl oz	64
Tomato	6 fl oz	33

VEGETABLES

Artichoke, cooked	1 medium	9
Asparagus	4 medium spears	16
Bean sprouts, stir fried	1/2 cup	10
Beans, snap, Italian, green and yellow	1/2 cup	6
Beets	1/2 cup sliced	5
Broccoli, raw	1/2 cup chopped	58
Brocolli, cooked	1/2 cup chopped	62
Brussels sprouts, cooked	1/2 cup	48
Cabbage, green, raw	1/2 cup shredded	20
Cabbage, green, cooked	1/2 cup shredded	22
Cabbage, red, raw	1/2 cup shredded	25

Vitamin C content of common foods cont'd

Cabage, red, cooked	1/2 cup shredded	31
Carrots, raw	1 (7-1/2" long x 1-1/8" diam)	7
Carrots, cooked	1/2 cup sliced	2
Cauliflower, raw	1/2 cup 1" pieces	36
Cauliflower, cooked	1/2 cup 1" pieces	34
Celery, raw	1 stalk (7-1/2" long)	2
Celery, cooked	1/2 cup diced	3
Chard, Swiss, cooked	1/2 cup chopped	16
Collards, cooked	1/2 cup choped	9
Corn, sweet, cooked	1 ear	5
Cucumber, raw	1/2 cup sliced	4
Greens, Mustard, cooked	1/2 cup chopped	18
Greens, Turnip, cooked	1/2 cup chopped	20
Kale, cooked	1/2 cup chopped	26
Kohlrabi	1/2 cup sliced	44
Lettuce, Iceberg	1 large leaf	1
Lettuce, Romaine or Kos	1/2 cup shredded	6
Okra, cooked	1/2 cup sliced	13
Parsnips, cooked	1/2 cup sliced	10
Peas, green, cooked	1/2 cup	11
Peas, Chinese pods, cooked	1/2 cup	38

Vitamin C content of common foods cont'd

Peppers, green & red, raw	1/2 cup chopped	64
Peppers green & red cooked	1/2 cup chopped	76
Peppers, hot chili, green & red, raw	1/2 cup chopped	182
Potatoes, baked, flesh and skin	1 medium (4-3/4" long)	26
Potatoes, flesh only	1 medium (4-3/4" long)	20
Potatoes, pared, boiled	1/2 cup	6
Radishes, raw	1/2 cup sliced	13
Rutabagas	1/2 cup cubed	18
Spinach, raw	1/2 cup chopped	8
Spinach, cooked	1/2 cup chopped	9
Squash, Summer, cooked	1/2 cup slices	5
Squash, Winter, cooked	1/2 cup cubes	10
Sweet potato, baked	1 (5" long)	28
Tomatoes, raw	1 medium (2-1/2" diam)	20
Tomatoes, cooked	1/2 cup	25
Turnips, cooked	1/2 cup	9

PREPARED FOODS

Coleslaw	1/2 cup	19

Source: Composition of Foods. Agriculture Handbook No.
8. US Department of Agriculture, Human Nutrition Information Service.

Note: In many cases a cooked serving of a vegetable contains
more vitamin C than a raw serving. This is because a cooked
vegetables usually pack more densely into a serving portion
(a cup for example) so in effect you get more weight of
vegetable per serving portion, hence more vitamin C.

The following appeared in the "Letters to the Editor" section of "Barron's" newspaper in June 94 when speculation was rampant that David Kessler, head of the Food and Drug Administration was drawing up plans to outlaw tobacco.

To the Editor:

I'm sure David Kessler's agency will take care of those lousy cigarettes and rid the nation of that dangerous drug nicotine.

After this problem has been eliminated, I certainly hope he will take a close look at ice cream and chocolate. Not a week passes when I have not been forced to observe, painful though it is, our younger generation jeopardizing its health by consuming these artery-clogging nightmares. These high-fat killers are responsible for millions of cancer and heart-attack deaths worldwide each year, and only dentists profit from their high sugar content. Anyone who has ever dabbled in ice cream or chocolate use knows how truly addictive these substances are. In fact, a recent survey of ice cream eaters found that 98% wanted to quit but couldn't.

My own grandfather continued to consume large quantities of German chocolate cake even after the arteries in his legs ceased to function and had to be replaced with synthetic ones. If ice cream and chocolate are recognized as addictive poisons, millions can be declared addicts and officially "disabled". They will become eligible to receive the federal financial support necessary to treat their addiction and save them from premature death.

George J. Piazza,
Meadowbrook, PA

6

Other Vitamins and Minerals That Can Help Smokers

There are a number of studies which indicate smokers have lower levels of other vitamins and minerals and a few also report protective benefits from taking supplements. There is less information to go on here, as fewer studies have been done in this area of research compared to the antioxidant nutrients in the previous chapters. Nevertheless you should make sure you get a sufficient intake of these vitamins and minerals by taking a daily multivitamin and mineral tablet.

Most multivitamin and mineral tablets contain the Recommended Dietary Allowance (RDA) of the B vitamins and several important minerals and this is what you need. A summary of the studies relevant to smokers is given below.

Dosage Measurement

In the chapter on vitamin C you were introduced to the unit of measure the gram (g), equal to about one twenty-eighth of an ounce. Then came the milligram (mg), equal to one thousandth of a gram. For some of the vitamins and minerals in this chapter we need an even smaller unit of measure, the microgram(mcg), equal to one millionth of a gram. So we have:

1 gram (g) = one twenty-eighth ounce (approx)

1 milligram (mg) = 1/1,000 gram

1 microgram (mcg) = 1/1,000,000 gram

Vitamin B12

The name Vitamin B12 is used to describe a group of water soluble compounds found only in foods of animal origin.

Several studies report vitamin B12 deficiency in both the blood and body tissue of smokers. Research indicates this is a result of vitamin B12 being used up in detoxifying the body of cyanide, one of the toxic components in cigarette smoke.

The Recommended Dietary Allowance (RDA) for vitamin B12 is 6 micrograms (mcg).

Folic Acid

Folic acid, also called folate, is a water soluble nutrient and member of the B vitamin group. It is an essential factor in the production of DNA, the genetic coding molecule. Smoking appears to cause a reduction of folate levels in blood serum and red blood cells.

A 1988 study of 73 male smokers showed that taking supplements of folate and vitamin B12 reduced the level of abnormal tissue in the lungs. Scientists believe abnormal lung tissue leads to lung cancer.

In a study in Spain in 1994, researchers found that smokers consistently showed lower folate intake and blood levels compared to non-smokers and at the end of their report stated that although quitting smoking is the best plan, for smokers who do not wish to give up the habit, increased folate intake could contribute to better health.

The Recommended Dietary Allowance for folic acid is 400 micrograms (mcg).

Women of Childbearing Age

The Centers for Disease Control, an arm of the US Department of Health and Human Services, issued the following recommendation in September 1992:

"All women of childbearing age in the United States who are capable of becoming pregnant should consume 400 micrograms (mcg) of folic acid per day for the purpose of reducing their risk of having a pregnancy affected with spina bifida or other NTDs (Neural Tube Defects)."

This is especially relevant to women smokers who are most likely at additional risk as a result of their tobacco habit.

The average consumption of dietary folic acid by American Women is only 200 micrograms (mcg), half the recommended amount.

Many good quality multivitamin and mineral tablets contain 400 micrograms (100% of the RDA) of folic acid, and this is the simplest way to ensure an adequate intake of this vitamin.

Vitamin B6

Vitamin B6 is an essential water soluble nutrient. It is required for the proper metabolism of proteins, fats and carbohydrates. Three studies show smokers may have lower blood levels of vitamin B6 than non-smokers.

The Recommended Dietary Allowance (RDA) for vitamin B6 is 2 milligrams (mg).

The Latest Survey Results

Data just released by the Department of Health and Human Services from their National Health and Nutrition Examination Survey show some sobering results. For Americans over the age of 50, the average intake of the three vitamins discussed above fell well below their respective RDA levels. A table giving these results is shown opposite.

Data for younger age groups and for smokers is not yet available but all indications point to similar if not poorer results.

Minerals

So far this book has dealt mainly with vitamin C, vitamin E and beta carotene which are all classed as antioxidant vitamins or more correctly antioxidant nutrients. The human body does however have two other major types of antioxidant defense systems.

Firstly the Antioxidant Enzymes - superoxide dismutase, catalase and glutathione peroxidase.

Secondly the Non-enzymatic Scavengers - uric acid, glutathione and thiols in proteins. These two groups of antioxidants also take an active part in defending cells from attack by free radicals and of major interest here are the antioxidant enzymes.

**Dietary Intake of Folic Acid, Vitamin B6 and Vitamin B12
Among Americans over 50**

Age	Folic Acid (mcg) RDA = 400	Vitamin B6 (mg) RDA = 2	Vitamin B12 (mcg) RDA = 6
50 - 59	231	1.51	3.55
60 - 69	249	1.57	3.68
70 - 79	243	1.51	3.04
80 and over	219	1.47	2.99

U.S. Department of Health and Human Services
Third National Health and Nutrition Examination Survey, Phase 1, 1988-91

Public Health Service, Centers for Disease Control and Prevention, National Center for Health Statistics

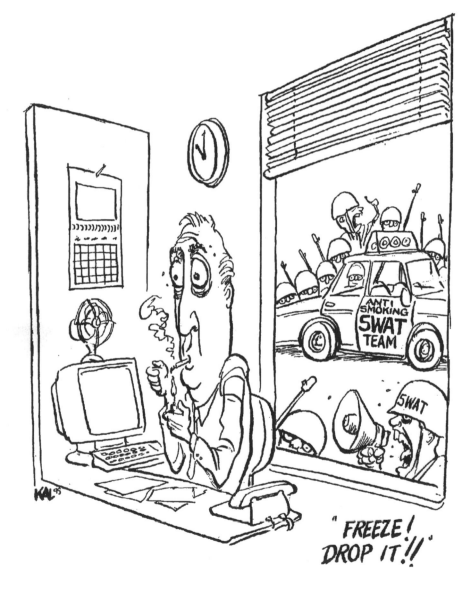

All other things being equal, the amount of antioxidant enzymes the body produces is largely determined by the genes you inherited from your parents, so there is an upper limit to this capacity. However a lack of certain essential minerals in your food can reduce the amount of these enzymes the body is able to produce, leading to a weakening of your defense systems. Taking a multivitamin and mineral supplement is good insurance against most deficiencies.

The important minerals required for the formation of the major antioxidant enzymes are shown below.

Selenium

It is known that selenium is an essential component in glutathione peroxidase a powerful member of the antioxidant enzyme family which helps reduce cell damage. It is also well accepted that selenium boosts the action of vitamin E.

There is conflicting evidence with regard to selenium levels in smokers, but a survey of studies suggests that smokers have lowered levels of selenium.

Some studies suggest selenium may play a role in the prevention of cancer and heart disease but the evidence is patchy.

There is no RDA for selenium but the Food and Nutrition Board of the National Academy of Sciences, gives the "Estimated Safe and Adequate Dose" for selenium as 70 microgams per day for adult males and 55 micrograms per day for adult females. Check your multivitamin tablet contains this mineral.

Warning:

Selenium can be toxic at doses above 200 mcg/day

Other Minerals

Zinc, copper and manganese are all essential building blocks in the formation of several antioxidant enzymes and should be present in your multivitamin and mineral tablet.

What to Take and How Much

What you are looking for is a multivitamin and mineral tablet or a B complex and mineral tablet which contains the following:

Vitamin B12	6 microgram (mcg)
Folic Acid	400 microgram (mcg)
Vitamin B6	2 milligram (mg)
Selenium	50-100 microgram (mcg)
Zinc	15 milligram (mg)
Copper	2-3 milligram (mg)
Manganese	2.5-5.0 milligram (mg)

Don't be too concerned if the multivitamin and mineral tablet you have found does not match these ingredients or doses exactly. Choose the tablet which comes closest. If it contains most, if not all, of these nutrients and roughly in the doses listed above, then you are well on your way to better nutrition than most smokers.

7

The Fruit and Vegetable Connection

One of the best health protection measures for smokers is to eat lots of fruit and vegetables. There is overwhelming evidence that a high intake of fruit and vegetables gives protection from cancer and heart disease, and provides many other health benefits.

The National Cancer Institute, the US Department of Agriculture, the US Department of Health and Human Services, the National Academy of Sciences and the American Health Foundation all recommend Americans eat five or more servings of fruit and vegetables every day as an important health protection measure.

Fruits and vegetables are rich sources of vitamin C, carotenes and dietary fiber, and scientists believe they may also contain other antioxidant micronutrients which protect from cancer and heart disease.

Are You Eating Yours ?

Results of a recent multi-state survey on the eating habits of over 23,000 Americans revealed some interesting data. Only 20% of the population consumed the recommended 5 or more daily servings of fruit and vegetables. This is hardly surprising considering the survey also revealed that only 8% of those questioned had heard of the "5-a-day" recommendation. The good news was that people who were aware of the program, had a higher consumption of fruit and vegetables.

What Is A Serving ?

Each of the following represents one serving. Fruits and vegetables can be fresh, dried, frozen or canned, they all count.

1/2 cup of fruit or vegetable (about 3-4 ounces)

3/4 cup of 100% juice (6 ounces)

1 cup of leafy greens

1/4 cup of dried fruit

1/2 cup of dried peas or beans

1 medium piece of fruit

The latest scientific studies show that drinking 2-1/2 cups of green or black tea gives the same health protection as one serving of fruit and vegetables.

Five-a-Day Is Easier Than You Think

Listed below are suggestions on how to get your servings of fruit and vegetables, try to include as many as you can in your daily diet.

Breakfast

● Drink a glass of fruit juice, fresh from your juicer or any 100% fruit juice.

● Eat a piece of fruit, orange and grapefruit are great, there are many others to choose from.

● Add sliced banana, pears, peaches, strawberries, raspberries or blueberries to your cereal. Don't forget in winter you can use dried fruits like raisins, apricots, peaches, prunes or figs.

● Have a bowl of fruit salad, you could use melon, peaches, pears, grapefruit, orange, pineapple, tangerines, kiwis, apple .... choose your favorites.

● Top your pancakes with fruit instead of syrup, try warm spiced apples in winter.

● Drink green or black tea

Breakfast on the run

● Take a banana, an apple or a bag of mixed dried fruit in the car with you, they're easy to eat on the move.

● Keep single serving cartons of fresh 100% juice in the refrigerator ready to grab and go.

● Order fresh orange juice from your fast food restaurant.

● Order tea as your hot beverage.

Lunch

● Have a salad or a soup that has vegetables.

● Chop up fresh vegetable sticks and eat with low-fat dip.

● Use your microwave to cook vegetables of your choice.

● Eat a piece of fruit like an apple, orange or a couple of plums or kiwis, your choice.

● Drink 100% fruit juice, hot or iced tea instead of soda.

Lunch on the run

● Use the soup and salad bar at your supermarket or fast food restaurant - choose a soup with vegetables.

● Many supermarkets have fresh cut, ready to eat fruit to go.

● Order a baked potato from your fast food restaurant.

● Order a salad or raw vegetables at your fast food restaurant.

Add lettuce, sprouts and tomatoes to your sandwich.

Add zucchini, carrot or celery sticks and a piece of fruit to your brown bag lunch.

Drink 100% fruit juice, or tea instead of a soda.

Dinner

● Many supermarkets have hot soups and a salad bar with food to go - don't forget the fresh cut ready to eat fruit.

Take home cleaned and sliced raw vegetables to cook or eat with a low-fat dip.

● You can now buy bags of ready prepared salads that will keep in your fridge for several days.

● Frozen vegetables and fruits are usually ready to cook.

Keep a stock of your favorite canned vegetables and fruits. Choose low salt vegetables and fruits in 100% fruit juice.

Wash and cut up carrots, celery, zucchini or jicama and keep them in the refrigerator, ready to cook or eat raw. Your vegetables can be kept fresh for days by keeping them wrapped in plastic.

Add vegetables to your main dish such as broccoli to your pasta or carrots to a casserole.

● Add raw vegetables or fruit to your green salad.

● Use fruits as a garnish on main dishes, apple or cranberry sauce or spiced apples or plain sliced fruit like peaches or melon.

● Order extra vegetables when you are eating out

● Drink 100% fruit juice instead of soda.

● Drink tea as your hot beverage.

Dessert

● Liven up a plain dessert with fresh fruit.

● Top your frozen yogurt with pineapple, papaya or any fruit of your choice.

● Serve fruit salad made with your favorite fruits - don't forget you can add dried fruits too for variety. In the winter add some spices and serve it warm.

● For a quick and easy dessert keep cans of fruit in your home - buy the ones packed in 100% fruit juice.

● Buy ready to eat chopped fruit at your supermarket.

● Add chopped fruit or berries to muffins, cakes or cookies or buy ready made.

If you like to snack

● Nibble on some grapes or raisins.

● Take along some dried fruit like apricots, prunes or figs.

● Drink a glass of 100% juice or hot or iced tea.

● Keep cut raw vegetables in water in the refrigerator.

● Keep a bowl of fresh fruit like grapes, apples, oranges, bananas etc. at arm's reach.

Microwave Your "5-A-DAY" (at work or at home)

Microwaving fruits and vegetables is easier than it looks. It saves a lot of time and they taste great! You don't even have to go to the market for fresh vegetables .... frozen vegetables can be microwaved too. Here are five simple rules to successfully microwaving produce.

1) For even cooking, cut into same-size pieces.
2) Stir, rearrange foods, or rotate a 1/2 turn, halfway through cooking.
3) Loosely cover foods so that steam can escape (use wax paper, plastic wrap or a vessel's lid)
4) Use a fork to pierce whole, unpeeled vegetables or fruits (like potatoes, yams, or apples) to keep them from bursting while cooking.
5) Let fruits and vegetables stand 3-5 minutes after microwaving to allow them to finish cooking.

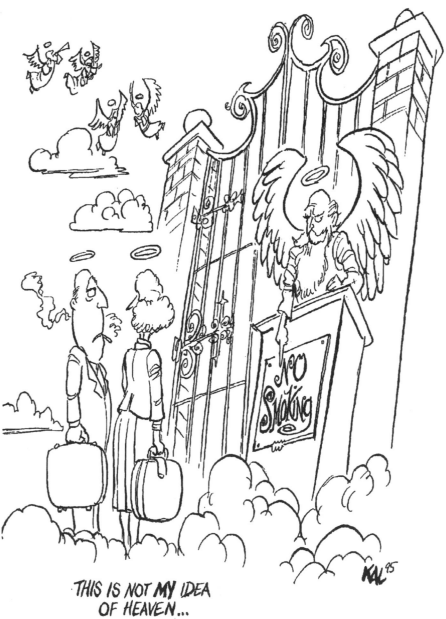

Microwave Guide for Single Servings or more (all cooking times on high setting)

Asparagus, Broccoli or Cauliflower - Arrange pieces in micro-safe dish (flowerettes or asparagus tips pointed towards center). Add 2 Tbsp. water, cover and cook.

1 cup	2-3 min
2 cup	3-4 min
1 lb (spears)	8-10 min

Brussels Sprouts - Peel away any wilted or brown outer layers. Arrange 1 pound in a 1-1/2 quart micro-safe dish and add 2 Tbsp. water, cover and cook.

1 cup	3-4 min
1 lb	6-7 min

Carrots - Trim stem and tops, slice. Place in micro-safe dish with 2 Tbsp. water, cover and cook.

3/4 cup	3-4 min
1-1/2 cup	4-5 min

Corn on the Cob - Peel husks back and remove silk, replace husks (if cooking more than one, arrange like "spokes" in the dish)

1 ear	3-4 min

Cut Corn or Peas (frozen) - Pour corn or peas into a micro-safe dish with 3 Tbsp. water, cover and cook.

1 cup	2-3 min
2 cup	4-5 min

Green Beans - Cut beans into 1" pieces and place in micro-safe dish with 1/4 cup water, cover and cook.

1 cup	3 min
1 lb	7-12 min

Greens - Rinse and coarsely chop greens. Place lightly wet leaves in micro-safe dish. Cover and cook.

    2 cups of leaves   2 min
    (makes 1/2 cup cooked)
    1-1/4 lb   7-10 min

Potato, Sweet Potato or Yam - Puncture a few times with a fork. Place on paper towel in microwave. Makes a good snack at work.

    1 medium   4-5 min
    2-3 min for each additional potato

Summer Squash (includes zucchini) - Trim off ends. Cut into 1/4" slices. Add 1/4 cup water to micro-safe dish, cover and cook.

    1-1/2 cup (sliced)   3-4 min
    1 lb   6-7 min

Winter Squash (Acorn, Hubbard, Banana, Danish and Spaghetti) - Cut into serving size pieces. Remove seeds and fibers. Place pieces cut side up in micro-safe dish. Sprinkle surface with 1/2 cup water or fruit juice. Cover and cook until tender when pierced with fork.

          10-13 min

8

Other Health Protection Measures for Smokers

Tea Drinking

The Japanese population has one of the highest rates of cigarette smoking but the lowest rate of lung cancer in the developed world. These facts had puzzled medical and scientific researchers for many years as it is widely accepted that smoking is one of the major risk factors for lung cancer. The most likely explanation is a dietary factor, as what people eat and drink has long been known to affect their cancer risk.

A favorite national beverage of the Japanese people is green tea, which they drink in large quantities, much like Americans drink coffee. For some time Japanese scientists had suspected that green tea was a cancer preventive and at least partly responsible for the low rates of lung cancer in Japanese smokers. Recent scientific studies have confirmed that a chemical known as epigallocatechin gallate (EGCG), one of the main constituents of green tea, lowers cholesterol and inhibits cancer growth.

● Researchers at the Laboratory for Cancer Research at Rutgers University in New Jersey ran an experiment on lung and stomach cancer in mice. Cancer causing chemicals were given to a large group of mice and half were given green tea as their only source of liquid and the other half water. Results showed that the mice receiving green tea had 60% less tumors than those receiving only water.

● Dr Fujiki, formerly of the National Cancer Center Research Institute in Tokyo, reported positive results on the antitumor effects of the green tea extract EGCG in a study in 1987. Noting that a Japanese tea-lover may consume about one gram of EGCG per day and taking this as proof that the chemical was non-toxic he decided to conduct a further research. His results showed strong anticancer activity in the stomach, liver and skin of mice. Dr Fujiki ended the report on the study results by stating: "We think that EGCG is a practical cancer chemopreventive agent to be implemented in daily life". He suggested the drinking of 5 cups of green tea every day as a good preventive measure for the general population. "Green tea cannot prevent every cancer," he added. "But it's the cheapest and most practical method for cancer prevention available to the general public".

● A research team at the American Health Foundation in Valhalla, NY showed that green tea could reduce the destructive effects of smoking. A chemical known as NNK, present in cigarette smoke, is believed to be one of the main factors in lung cancer development in smokers. Mice given green tea and exposed to NNK had only half the lung tumors of mice given only water. The mice given green tea did not gain as much weight as the untreated group but otherwise no ill effects were seen.

● Results from several studies also reveal that drinking four or more cups of tea per day lowers the risk of artery clogging and heart disease.

● Recent research by Dr John Weisburger at the American Health Foundation has revealed that black tea has anti-cancer and heart disease prevention effects as strong as those of green tea. His laboratory experiments reveal antioxidant substances in black tea similar to those found in green tea and showing the same health protection benefits.

Weisburger believes that drinking five cups of any green or black tea per day provides similar protective benefits to eating two servings of vegetables. He also adds that for the so called "herbal teas", there is no evidence at this time that they show any protection against heart disease or cancer.

What to Drink

There has been much research work done on green tea and its health protection properties are well established and accepted by a large section of the scientific community. This has come about simply because of the interest of Japanese and Chinese scientists in their national beverage. Green tea is available in health food stores and many of the major food chains. Many Chinese restaurants serve green tea.

For black tea the scientific evidence on its ability to protect from heart disease and cancer is not as well documented compared to green tea, but the gap is closing fast as more and more studies are completed. For now a good choice is green tea, but if it is not to your liking, or you have trouble finding it, then black tea is fine. Black tea is available almost everywhere and is the most common tea served in the United States, Canada, UK, Ireland, South Africa, Latin America and the Near East.

Eating Fish May Protect Smoker's Lungs

The July 28th, 1994 issue of the New England Journal of Medicine reported the results of a study by medical researchers at the University of Minnesota School of Public Health. The report concluded that a high dietary intake of omega-3 fatty acids, found mainly in fish, may protect cigarette smokers from bronchitis and emphysema.

Scientists have noted for years that polyunsaturated fatty acids, abundant in fish, help relieve chronic inflammatory diseases such as rheumatoid arthritis and ulcerative colitis.

Both chronic bronchitis and emphysema, two of the major diseases which affect smokers, are thought to start with chronic inflammation of the lung. This lead researchers to study the effects of eating fish on smoker's risk of lung disease.

The research team interviewed 8,960 current or former smokers from four separate areas of the US, Forsyth County North Carolina; Jackson, Mississippi; the suburbs of Minneapolis; and Washington County, Maryland. Average consumption of fish during the previous year for each participant was assessed using a dietary questionnaire. All members of the group were examined by a team of physicians and cases of emphysema and bronchitis noted.

Results revealed that individuals eating an average of four servings of fish per week cut their risk of bronchitis or emphysema by 45% compared to those eating only half a serving per week.

The researchers believe fish oil, which contains omega-3 fatty acids, inhibits inflammation and deterioration of lung tissue in smokers.

How Much Fish Do You Need to Eat

The serving sizes used in the study were as follows:

Canned Tuna fish	3-4 oz (85-113 gram)
Dark Meat Fish (eg. salmon, mackerel, swordfish, sardines and bluefish)	3-5 oz (85-142 gram)
Other fish (eg cod, perch, catfish)	3-5 oz (85-142 gram)

Although this one study does not prove that eating fish will protect you from bronchitis and emphysema, several other studies support the theory.

● The Department of Health and Human Services conducts a National Health and Nutrition Examination Survey every ten years to find out what Americans eat and their state of health. An examination of data from the latest survey showed a link between a high intake of fish and low rates of bronchitis.

● In a study of telephone workers in the United States and Japan, researchers found the Japanese had lower rates of chronic bronchitis than Americans despite the fact both groups smoked the same number of cigarettes per day.

A possible explanation - the Japanese diet is high in fish intake, whereas the American diet is low.

What About Supplements

Omega-3 fatty acids, also called omega-3 polyunsaturated fatty acids are also available in supplement form, usually as gelcaps. However as scientists are unsure at this time whether it is the omega-3 fatty acids in fish which appear to give protection or some other as yet unknown component of fish your best policy is to eat the fish.

If you don't like fish or can't eat four or more servings per week then supplements are another option. One serving of fish provides about 125 milligrams (mg) of omega-3 polyunsaturated fatty acids.

9

The "Quit Smoking" Option

Although the main thrust of this book deals with ways you can reduce the health risks of smoking, quitting smoking is certainly the best health protection measure you can take.

No doubt you have heard preachings about the "evils of tobacco" more times than you care to remember and don't need to hear any more. This author agonized for many a long hour as to whether to include this chapter. Eventually however, it was decided that a book about smoking and health would not be complete without some information on how to quit. If you are not interested in quitting, this is a free country, you are perfectly at liberty to stop reading right here and concentrate on the health protection measures in the rest of the book.

If you are serious about quitting, there are several groups and organizations which can help. Their names, addresses and phone numbers are listed on the following pages.

Quitting smoking is easy !

I know, I've done it hundreds of times.

American Heart Association

They provide an information package which contains two booklets titled "Calling It Quits". The first deals with making a plan of how you are going to quit. The second goes over ways of coping with the urge to start again. It shows examples of everyday situations where the pressure to smoke is strong and gives suggestions of how best to cope with them.

This is all solid, useful information, and it is easy to understand and follow the directions given. A simple no-nonsense guide which will be useful to all smokers. Call and they will mail you their free information pack.

TEL 800 242 8721

American Lung Association

Calling the 800 number listed below will connect you with your American Lung Association local office. They will send you a free "Quit Kit" which has the following brochures:

"Questions and Answers about Smoking"
"Nicotine Addiction and Cigarettes"
"What Happens When a Smoker Quits"
"Tips for Weight Control "

plus a brochure and order form for their "Freedom from Smoking for You and Your Family". This a comprehensive 54 page guide to quitting smoking for which they charge a nominal sum.

The American Lung Association also offers a "Freedom From Smoking" course for which they charge about $100. This is a group program with seven sessions over a seven week period for those who need outside help to quit.

The information and "quit smoking" programs offered by each local office may vary, call for details.

TEL 800 492 7527

American Cancer Society

This community-based voluntary health organization will send you several brochures on quitting smoking. These include "Smart Move, a Stop Smoking Guide" and " The Most Often Questions About Smoking, Tobacco, and Health ... and the Answers."

For those who would like some help to quit, ACS runs a program called "Freshstart". About 12 to 15 persons form a quit smoking group and are led by a trained ex-smoker. The program consists of four one-hour sessions held during a two-week period. There is no charge for the program. Call for details.

TEL 800 ACS 2345.

Seventh-day Adventists

There are a large number of Adventist hospitals throughout the country which are actively involved in health education and many run "quit smoking" programs.

Their most up-to-date program called "Breathe Free: The Plan to Stop Smoking" is user friendly, research based and gives support through the three stages of smoking cessation: preparation, breaking free and maintenance. The program consists of nine sessions, each one and a half to two hours long, spread over a one month period. Programs in some areas may charge a fee, usually in the range $30 - $60.

A two-year study by Loma Linda University found that after one year, 65% of smokers who completed the program remained cigarette free. Results may however vary depending on the skill of the program conductor and the level of commitment of the participants.

During the last 30 years, worldwide Adventist programs have helped over 20 million people stop smoking. Look in the Yellow Pages telephone book under "hospitals" or "churches" for a Seventh-day Adventist or Adventists listing.

Office on Smoking and Health

The Office on Smoking and Health (OSH) is an arm of the federal government's Department of Health and Human Services. They offer the following smoking cessation publications:

"Clearing the Air: How to Quit Smoking and Quit for Keeps", a 24 page guide with a comprehensive list of tips on quitting smoking.

"Out of the Ashes: Choosing a Method to Quit Smoking", a 16 page booklet designed to help you choose a quit smoking method. Covers self-help, advice from your doctor, nicotine chewing gum, nicotine patch, group approaches, conditioning methods, live-in programs, hypnosis, acupuncture and over-the-counter products.

"The Health Benefits of Smoking Cessation: At a Glance", a 4 page pamphlet highlighting the specific benefits of quitting smoking.

"Good News for Smokers 50 and Older", a fact sheet outlining the health benefits of quitting smoking for those over 50.
You can obtain these publications by writing to:

Office on Smoking and Health
Mail Stop K-50
4770 Buford Highway, NE
Atlanta
GA 30341-3714

or you can telephone (404) 488 5707. You will be connected to a voicemail system, press 2 and ask for "quit smoking" booklets. Be sure to allow 3-6 weeks for delivery.

Yellow pages

Listed in the Yellow Pages telephone book under the heading "smokers" or "smoking" you will find the names and numbers of various commercial enterprises which are set up to help smokers to quit. These companies or individual therapists charge a fee. Services include such things as acupunture, hypnosis, psychotherapy etc.

Several well conducted surveys reveal that 90% of smokers quit without any outside help other than information booklets, support from friends or the advice of their doctor or other health professional. This being the case you are well advised to start with the "free" services listed above. Having said this, some people who find it difficult to quit on their own do succeed with the help of commercial programs.

After you have quit smoking

Quitting smoking is the best step you can take to protect your health. It reduces your risk of cancer, heart disease and several other smoking related ailments by a large margin.

You should however be aware, that when you quit, your risk does not drop to the same low level as a lifetime nonsmoker. It will be several years before your risk profile gets down to that area. For this reason it makes good sense to continue with the health protection measures given in this book even after you quit.

10

Smoking, Nutrition and Politics -
or why you probably haven't heard about
health protection for smokers before

The scientific community is reluctant to tell smokers
about any health protection given by fruits and vegetables
and antioxidant nutrients. They fear that broadcasting this
information will lead smokers to lessen their efforts to quit
smoking, which is the number one public health policy
directed at smokers.

To a limited extent this is a genuine fear as there is always
the possibility that some smokers will adopt the attitude "I
don't have to worry about the health risks of smoking, I eat
lots of fruits and vegetables and take vitamins".

However the downside of limiting the public's knowledge of antioxidant nutrients is that the great majority of smokers are deprived of the health protection benefits available. Obviously having written this book the author believes smokers have the right to know the whole story about antioxidant vitamins and the health protection they can offer.

Drug Companies

The majority of the large drug companies do not promote vitamins heavily because there is little profit to be made. Vitamins have been around for years and are non patentable. They are cheap to manufacture and sell at low prices, providing little incentive to advertise and promote them.

There are of course exceptions, one or two of the drug giants take vitamins seriously, believe in their health benefits and promote them vigorously. A good example is chemical and drugs giant Hoffmann-LaRoche. Impressed with reports from studies on beta carotene and anticipating increased demand they have just built a new production plant in Freeport, Texas. When fully operational it will produce 350 tons of beta carotene a year, enough to supply every American adult with a 10,000 IU (6 mg) capsule every day.

A few drug companies have synthesized compounds with roughly the same properties as the antioxidant vitamins, but so far these patented compounds have had little impact on the marketplace.

Doctors

A recent survey showed only 10% of doctors had any training in nutrition at medical school. Of those who had training, 75% said it was inadequate and involved less than a total of 40 hours spread over a 5 year course of study. Few doctors are a reliable source of information on nutrition or vitamins.

Again there are exceptions, some doctors have an excellent knowledge of nutrition, usually acquired on their own initiative, but unfortunately they are few and far between. After medical school they are usually too busy to learn about the latest findings in preventive medicine, a not very fashionable subject.

A great deal of the information on new drugs or new uses for old drugs comes from the promotional and marketing literature of big drug companies and little or no information about vitamins reaches doctors by this route. There is plenty of information published on nutrition but few doctors have the time to keep up with the latest developments. Most confine their reading to the medical journals, the New England Journal of Medicine, Journal of the American Medical Association, Lancet, etc. In this age of information overload it is just impossible for them, or indeed anyone but specialists in nutrition and disease prevention, to stay current.

It is also the case that doctors do not expect you to come to their offices and say "How do I stay healthy ", people only visit when they are sick. Patients are partly to blame for this situation but doctors do not encourage patients to visit their offices on this basis, as most of their training is aimed at treating illness when it arises, not preventing it.

Indeed it is a sad fact but true, that the healthcare system we have in the U.S. expends most of its time and energy treating us when we become ill rather than trying to prevent illness before it occurs. This system now has a life of its own, has grown to enormous proportions and is very much set in its ways. Changing the attitudes, beliefs and direction of the medical profession towards preventive medicine, in which nutrition and vitamins play a large role, promises to be a slow process. Fortunately, most Americans realize this is the direction which must be taken if sharply rising medical care costs are to be brought under control.

As a final point it must be remembered that nutrition and vitamin research has been considered flaky, quackery, oddball and not worthy of serious attention for decades. It is only in the last 10 years or so that it has become respectable, and for many in the healthcare industry old ideas die hard.

The Media

Over the years, the media - TV, Radio, newspapers and magazines - have provided a wealth of information on nutrition and health protection. Indeed they are probably responsible for the greater part of the knowledge most people have in this area. Results from the latest scientific studies and surveys on health and nutrition are regularly and usually accurately reported.

Occasionally the time or number of column inches devoted to a story does not allow a comprehensive or well-balanced review of the subject matter and there is the usual media tendency towards over-dramatization, but for the most part they cover the subject well. Books especially are very strong in the nutrition/health subject area. You can find almost any information your heart could desire from the wealth of titles already published and new titles appear almost daily.

The Food and Drug Administration (FDA)

The FDA regulates new drugs entering the market place, ensures the quality of all manufactured drugs and protects the population from unsafe medicines.

To have a new drug approved or an old drug approved for a new use requires extensive testing costing upwards of $100 million per drug and takes on average 10 years to complete. Since there is no big money to be made from vitamins it follows that no drug company will submit any vitamin for FDA testing.

Many leading researchers in the nutrition field believe the FDA is stuck with the 40 year old view that vitamins are necessary only to prevent deficiency diseases and will not accept the vital role they play in disease prevention and the maintenance of optimum health.

Recently however, the FDA has officially recognized that smokers have a greater need for vitamin C than nonsmokers. The RDA for vitamin C for smokers has been raised to 100mg per day, whereas the RDA for nonsmokers is 60mg per day. Hopefully this is only a first step the right direction.

Health Authorities

You may wonder why you don't hear about the health benefits of vitamins from health authorities? Well you do if you listen carefully.

Leading health authorities, the National Academy of Sciences, the US Department of Agriculture's Food and Nutrition Service, the American Health Foundation and the National Cancer Institute recommend all Americans eat at least five and preferably more servings of fruits and vegetables every day. Fruits and vegetables are the main food sources of carotenes and vitamin C.

Unfortunately the advertising budget to promote such healthy eating habits is small. In 1993 the National Cancer Institute spent $400,000 to promote its "Better Health" campaign. Compare this to Kellogg who in 1992 spent $34 million to promote "Frosted Flakes."

11

Summing It All Up

The Risks and What You Can Do About Them

If you smoke there is little doubt you are at increased risk from a wide range of health complaints and that the best policy is to quit.

However as federal government statistics show, 46 million Americans, about 25% of the adult population, still choose to smoke. If you are one of this group then there are many steps you can take to reduce the risks and protect your health.

You should also bear in mind that even if you quit today you will remain at increased health risk for several years as a result of your smoking history. This being the case it is wise to continue with as many of the health protection measures as you can after you quit.

Antioxidant Vitamins and Your Diet

Changing your diet, taking vitamin supplements or a combination of the two is a good way to reduce the health risks. There is overwhelming evidence linking a high intake of the antioxidant vitamins C, E and beta carotene or foods rich in these antioxidants with reduced risk of heart disease, cancer, especially of the lung and cataracts. These are precisely the diseases most likely to affect smokers.

Numerous food consumption surveys and laboratory tests show that smokers are particularly at risk as they have a low intake and lower blood and tissue levels of these essential vitamins.

Several health authorities recommend the consumption of at least five and preferably more servings of fruit and vegetables every day as a protection against heart disease and cancer. This is sound policy as it will provide you with increased amounts of vitamin C and carotenes. Furthermore scientists believe fruits and vegetables most likely contain other as yet unidentified health promoting compounds, especially antioxidants, which may give protection from disease.

However, if you can't reach this recommended intake of fruit and vegetables then taking supplements is a sound way to bring your vitamin intake up to levels which ensure better health.

Since the protection from heart disease linked to a high intake of vitamin E appears only at intakes well above those obtainable from diet, supplements are the only realistic way to get this vitamin.

Other Vitamins and Minerals

There is some evidence that smokers are deficient in certain B vitamins and some minerals so taking a multivitamin and mineral tablet to make sure you get an adequate supply of these nutrients makes good sense.

If you don't follow any of the other health protection strategies in this book then at least take a multivitamin and mineral tablet. It is the easiest health protection step you can take. Most multivitamin tablets will give you some vitamin C, vitamin E and beta carotene plus the B vitamins and a good selection of minerals. It is a sound first step to health protection for smokers.

Drinking Tea

For green tea the evidence that it acts as a cancer preventive is strong. Several Japanese and Chinese researchers have found in laboratory experiments that it has strong cancer inhibiting properties and studies of populations who drink a lot of this tea tend to confirm these findings. Several researchers recommend green tea wholeheartedly to everyone as an inexpensive and readily available cancer preventive. Whether you actually like the taste of green tea is a matter of personal preference, but it is well worth giving it a try.

The evidence from population studies that black tea protects from cancer and heart disease is thin. However there is an extensive database of laboratory work which shows anti-cancer and anti-heart disease properties. Black tea is widely available in both regular and decaffinated varieties, with beneficial antioxidant levels similar to green tea.

Eating Fish

There are limited data on eating fish as a protective measure for smokers but this is a measure you can include with little effort.

The Best Strategy

Listed below are the health protection measures for smokers discussed in the book. They are ranked in approximate order of importance, most important first. The only advice we would offer here is do the best you can. If you can manage one or two, that's great, three or four, even better. The more of these health protection measures you can include in your lifestyle the greater the contribution to your health. Use as many of them as you can, you don't have to include them all at once.

● Increase your intake of fruit and vegetables to five or more servings per day.

● Take supplements of vitamin C and beta carotene if your fruit and vegetable intake doesn't reach at least 5 servings per day.

● Take a vitamin E supplement

● Take a multivitamin and mineral supplement

● Drink tea, either green or black.

● Eat more fish

Here's wishing you a long and healthy life !

References

Listed on the following pages are references for all the studies from which this book was put together. There is a lot of material here and no doubt very few people will read it all. However a quick look will give you some idea of the number of studies involved, the hundreds of scientists from all over the world who conducted them, and the enormous amount of work they put in. Smoking, nutrition and disease prevention have been study areas which have received an great deal of attention over the last twenty years.

How references are listed

Most references listed here come from scientific journals such as the "Journal of the American Medical Association" or the "American Journal of Clinical Nutrition" to give two examples. These journals are usually published monthly and are basically magazines in which scientists announce the results of their studies. Competition to get studies published is stiff and only the best or most interesting are published. A typical reference is published below and is followed by an explanation of meaning of the various terms used.

Willett W et al. Relation of serum vitamins A and E and carotenoids to the risk of cancer. New England Journal of Medicine 310:430-434, 1984

"Willett W" - The head researcher's last name is "Willett" and first initial "W".

"et al" - This is a shorthand phrase used to indicate that more than one scientist took part in the study but to save space the other names are not listed.

"Relation of serum vitamins A and E and carotenoids to the risk of cancer" - this is the topic of the research.

New England Journal of Medicine 310:430-434, 1984 - The results of the study were published in the "New England Journal of Medicine" in volume 310 and covered pages 430 to 434. The results were published in 1984.

Chapter 3: Beta Carotene and Your health.

How Beta Carotene Works
Foote CS et al. Quenching singlet oxygen. Annals of the New York Academy of Sciences 171:139-148, 1970.

Are You Getting Enough Beta Carotene
National Academy of Sciences. Diet, nutrition and cancer. Washington DC; National Academy Press 1982.

US Department of Agriculture / US Department of Health and Human Services. Nutrition and your health. Dietary Guidelines for Americans. Washington DC: US Government Printing Office 1980.

US Department of Health and Human Services, National Cancer Institute, National Institutes of Health. Diet, nutrition and cancer prevention: A guide to food choices (NIH publication no 85-2711) Washington DC: US Government printing Office, 1984.

US Department of Agriculture, Nationwide food consumption survey (report 86-1). Washington DC: US Government Printing Office, 1987.

US Department of Agriculture. Continuing survey of food intake by individuals (report no 85-3). Washington DC: US Government Printing Office, 1987.

Lachance P. Dietary Intake of Carotenes and the Carotene Gap. Clinical Nutrition 7:118-122, 1988.

Smoking and Beta Carotene
Witter FR et al. Folate, carotene and smoking. American Journal of Obstetrics and Gynecology 144:857, 1982.

Davis C et al. Relation between cigarette smoking and serum vitamin A and carotene in candidates for the Lipid Research Clinics Coronary Prevention Trial. American Journal of Epidemiology 118:445, 1983.

Russel-Briefel R et al. The relationship of plasma carotenoids to health and biochemical factors in middle- aged men. American Journal of Epidemiology 122:741-749, 1985.

Chow CK et al. Lower levels of vitamin C and carotenes in plasma of cigarette smokers. Journal of the American College of Nutrition 5:305-312, 1986.

Stryker WS et al. The relation of diet, cigarette smoking and alcohol consumption to plasma beta carotene and alpha-tocopherol levels. American Journal of Epidemiology 127:283-296, 1988.

Carotenes and Lung Cancer
Bjelke E . Dietary vitamin A and lung cancer. International Journal of Cancer 15:561-565, 1975.

MacLennan R et al. Risk factors for lung cancer in Singapore Chinese, a population with high female incidence rate. International Journal of Cancer 20:854-860, 1977.

Hirayama T. Diet and cancer. Nutrition and Cancer 1:67-81, 1979.

Mettlin C et al. Vitamin A and lung cancer. Journal of the National Cancer Institute 62:1435-1438, 1979.

Gregor A et al. Comparison of dietary histories in lung cancer cases and controls with special reference to vitamin A. Nutrition and Cancer 2:93-97, 1980.

Shekelle R et al. Dietary vitamin A and risk of cancer in the Western Electric study. Lancet 2:1185-1189, 1981

Kvale G et al. Dietary habits and lung cancer risk. International Journal of Cancer 32:397-405 1983.

Hinds M et al. Dietary vitamin A, carotene, vitamin C and risk of lung cancer in Hawaii. American Journal of Epidemiology 119:227-237, 1984.

Willett W et al. Relation of serum vitamins A and E and carotenoids to the risk of cancer. New England Journal of Medicine 310:430-434, 1984.

Samet JM et al. Lung cancer risk and vitamin A consumption in New Mexico. American Review of Respiratory Disease 131:198-202, 1985.

Wu AH et al. Smoking and other risk factors for lung cancer in women. Journal of the National Cancer Institute 74:747- 751, 1985.

Nomura AM et al. Serum vitamin levels and the risk of cancer of specific sites in Hawaiian males of Japanese ancestry. Cancer Research 45:2369-2372, 1985.

Menkes M et al. Serum beta carotene, vitamins A and E, selenium, and the risk of lung cancer. New England Journal of Medicine 315:1250-1254, 1986.

Pisani P et al. Carrots, green vegetables and lung cancer: A case control study. International Journal of Epidemiology 15:463-468, 1986.

Ziegler R et al. Carotenoid intake, vegetables and the risk of lung cancer among white men in New Jersey. American Journal of Epidemiology 123:1080-1091, 1986.

Bond GG et al. Dietary vitamin A and lung cancer: results of a case control study among chemical workers. Nutrition and Cancer 9:109-121 1987.

Byers TE et al. Diet and lung cancer risk: Findings from the Western New York diet study. American Journal of Epidemiology 125:351-363, 1987.

Gey KF et al. Plasma levels of antioxidant vitamins in relation to ischemic heart disease and cancer. American Journal of Clinical Nutrition 45:1368-1377, 1987.

Humble CG et al. Use of quantified and frequency indices of vitamin A intake in a case-control study of lung cancer. International Journal of Epidemiology 16:341-346, 1987.

Kromhout D. Essential micronutrients in relation to carcinogenesis. American Journal of Clinical Nutrition 45:1361-1367, 1987.

Paganinni-Hill A et al. Vitamin A, beta carotene and the risk of cancer: a prospective study. Journal of the National Cancer Institute 79:443-448, 1987.

Pastorini U et al. Vitamin A and female lung cancer: a case-control study on plasma and diet. Nutrition and Cancer 10:171-179, 1987.

Fontham ETH et al. Dietary vitamins A and C and lung cancer risk in Louisiana. Cancer 62:2267-2273, 1988.

Holst PA et al. For debate: pet birds as an independent risk factor for lung cancer. British Medical Journal 297:1319-1321, 1988.

Koo LC. Dietary habits and lung cancer risk among Chinese females in Hong Kong who never smoked. Nutrition and Cancer 11:155-172, 1988.

Wald NJ et al. Serum beta carotene and subsequent risk of cancer: results from a BUPA study. British Journal of Cancer 57:428-433, 1988.

Kune GA et al. Serum levels of beta carotene, vitamin A, and zinc in male lung cancer cases and controls. Nutrition and Cancer 12:169-176, 1989.

Mettlin C. Milk drinking, other beverage habits and lung cancer risk. International Journal of Cancer 43:608- 612, 1989.

LeMarchand L et al. Vegetable consumption and lung cancer risk: a population-based case-control study in Hawaii. Journal of the National Cancer Institute 81:1158-1164, 1989.

Connet JE et al. Relationship between carotenoids and cancer: the Multiple Risk Factor Intervention Trial (MRFIT) study. Cancer 64:126-134, 1989.

Stahelin HB et al. Beta carotene and cancer prevention: the Basel Study. American Journal of Clinical Nutrition 53:265S-269S, 1991.

LeMarchand L et al. Intake of specific carotenoids and lung cancer risk. Cancer Epidemiology, Biomarkers & Prevention 2(3):183-187, 1993.

Heinonen OP et al. The effect of vitamin E and beta carotene on the incidence of lung cancer and other cancers in male smokers. New England Journal of Medicine 330:15:1029-1035, 1994.

Carotenes and Heart Disease
Rimm EB et al. Vitamin E consumption and the risk of coronary heart disease in men. New England Journal of Medicine 328:1450-1456, 1993.

Morris DL et al. Serum carotenoids and heart disease. Journal of the American Medical Association 272:18:1439-1441, 1994.

Kardinaal AFM et al. Antioxidants in adipose tissue and the risk of myocardial infarction: the EURAMIC study. Lancet 342:1379-1384, 1993

Carotenes and Cataract
Langseth L. Preserving precious sight. Antioxidant Vitamins Newsletter No6:3, July 1993 (editorial).

Taylor A. Cataract: Relationships between nutrition and oxidation. Journal of the American College of Nutrition 12:2, 138-146, 1993.

Christen WG et al. A Prospective study of cigarette smoking and risk of cataract in men. Journal of the American Medical Association 268:8 989-993, 1992.

Hankinson SE et al. A Prospective study of cigarette smoking and risk of cataract in women. Journal of the American Medical Association 268:8 994-998, 1992.

West S. Does the smoke get in your eyes? Journal of the American Medical Association 268:8 1025-1026, 1992.

Jacques PF et al. Epidemiologic evidence of a role for the antioxidant vitamins and carotenoids in cataract prevention. American Journal of Clinical Nutrition 53:352S- 355S, 1991.

Knekt P et al. Serum antioxidant vitamins and risk of cataract. British Medical Journal 305:1392-1394, 1992.

Mouth and Throat Cancer
Garewal H. Potential role of beta carotene in prevention of oral cancer. American Journal of Clinical Nutrition 53:294S-297S, 1991.

Garewal H et al. Response of oral leukoplakia to beta carotene. Journal of Clinical Oncology 8:10:1715-1720, 1990.

Breast and Gynecological Cancers
Gaby SK et al. Vitamin Intake and Health, Marcel Dekker Inc, 1991.

Wald NJ et al. Plasma retinol, beta carotene, and vitamin E levels in relation to the future risk of breast cancer. British Journal of Cancer 49:321-324, 1984.

Willett W et al. Relation of serum vitamins A and E and carotenoids to the risk of cancer. New England Journal of Medicine 310:430-434, 1984.

LaVecchia C et al. Dietary factors and the risk of breast cancer. Nutrition and Cancer 10:205-214, 1987.

Katsouyanni K et al. Risk of breast cancer among Greek women in relation to nutrient intake. Cancer 61:181-185, 1988.

Rohan TE et al. A population-based case-control study of diet and breast cancer in Australia. American Journal of Epidemiology 128:478-489, 1988.

Marubini E et al. The relationship of dietary intake and serum levels of retinol and beta carotene with breast cancer: results of a case control study. Cancer 61:173- 180, 1988.

Marshall JR et al. Diet and smoking in the epidemiology of cancer of the cervix. Journal of the National Cancer Institute 70:847-851, 1983.

LaVecchia C et al. Dietary vitamin A and the risk of invasive cervical cancer International Journal of Cancer 34:319-322, 1984.

Wylie-Rossett JA et al. Influence of vitamin A on cervical dysplasia and carcinoma in situ. Nutrition and Cancer 6:49- 57, 1984.

Brock K et al. Nutrients in diet and plasma and risk of in situ cervical cancer. Journal of the National Cancer Institute 80:580-585, 1988.

Verreault R et al. A case-control study of diet and invasive cervical cancer. International Journal of Cancer 43:1050-1054, 1989.

Hirayama T. Diet and cancer. Nutrition and Cancer 1:67- 81,1979

Orr JW et al. Corpus and cervix cancer: A nutritional comparison. American Journal of Obstetrics and Gynecology 153:775-779, 1985.

LaVecchia C et al. Nutrition and diet in the etiology of endometrial cancer. Cancer 57:1248-1253, 1986.

How Safe is Beta Carotene
Bendich A. The safety of beta carotene. Nutrition and Cancer 11: 207-214, 1988.

Mathews-Roth MM. Beta carotene therapy for Erythropoietic Protoporphyria and other photosensitivity diseases. Biochimie 68:875-884, 1986

Odds and Ends
Aoki K et al. Smoking, alcohol drinking and serum carotenoid levels. Japanese Journal of Cancer Research (Gann) 78:1049-1056, 1987.

Micozzi MS et al. Plasma carotenoid response to chronic intake of selected foods and beta carotene supplements in men. American Journal of Clinical Nutrition 55:1120-1125, 1992.

Coeyman M. New plant feeds vitamin hunger. Chemical Week November 10, 1993.

Sources of Beta Carotene
Micozzi M et al. Carotenoid analyses of selected raw and cooked foods associated with lower risk of cancer. Journal of the National Cancer Institute 82:282-285, 1990.

Mangels AR et al. Carotenoid content of fruits and vegetables: An evaluation of data. Journal of the American Dietetic Association 93:284-296, 1993.

Chapter 4: Vitamin E and Smoker's Health.

Are You Getting Enough Vitamin E
Murphy SP et al. Vitamin E intakes and sources in the United States. American Journal of Clinical Nutrition 52:361-367, 1990

Smoking and Vitamin E
Cade JE et al. Relationship between diet and smoking - is the diet of smokers different? Journal of Epidemiology and Community Health 45:270-272, 1991.

Pacht ER et al. Deficiency of vitamin E in the alveolar fluid of cigarette smokers. Journal of Clinical Investigation 77:789-796, 1986.

Myamoto H et al. Serum selenium and vitamin E concentrations in families of lung cancer patients. Cancer 60:1159-1162, 1987.

Vitamin E and Protection From Heart Disease
Reducing the Health Consequences of Smoking: 25 Years of Progress, a Report of the Surgeon General, 1989. US Dept of Health and Human Services.

Stampfer MJ et al. Vitamin E consumption and the risk of coronary heart disease in women. New England Journal of Medicine 328:1444-1449, 1993.

Rimm EB et al. Vitamin E consumption and the risk of coronary heart disease in men. New England Journal of Medicine 328:1450-1456, 1993.

Gey KF et al. Plasma levels of antioxidant vitamins in relation to ischemic heart disease and cancer. American Journal of Clinical Nutrition 45:1368-1377, 1987.

Verlangieri AJ et al. Effects of d-alpha-tocopherol supplementation on experimentally induced primate atherosclerosis. Journal of the American College of Nutrition 11:2, 131-138, 1992.

Vitamin E and Protection for the Lungs
Pacht ER et al. Deficiency of vitamin E in the alveolar fluid of cigarette smokers. Journal of Clinical Investigation 77:789-796, 1986.

Mayamoto H et al. Serum selenium and vitamin E concentrations in families of lung cancer patients. Cancer 60:1159-1162, 1987.

Menkes MS et al. Serum beta carotene, vitamins A and E, selenium, and the risk of lung cancer. New England Journal of Medicine 315:1250-1254, 1986.

Mouth, Throat and Esophageal Cancer
Gridley G et al. Vitamin supplement use and reduced risk of oral and pharyngeal cancer. American Journal of Epidemiology 135:1083-1092.

Tuyns AJ et al. Nutrition and cancer of the esophagus. In "Diet and Human Carcinogenesis", Elsevier Science Publishers, New York, pp 71-79, 1985.

Vitamin E and Cataract
Jacques PF et al. Epidemiologic evidence of a role for the antioxidant vitamins and carotenoids in cataract prevention. American Journal of Clinical Nutrition 53:352S- 355S, 1991.

Knekt P et al. Serum antioxidant vitamins and risk of cataract. British Medical Journal 305:1392-1394, 1992.

Jacques PF et al. Antioxidant status in persons with and without senile cataract. Archives of Opthalmology 106:337- 340, 1988.

Gastrointestinal Cancer
Mergens WJ et al. Alpha tocopherol: uses in preventing nitrosamine formation. In "Environmental Aspects of N-nitroso Compounds. IARC Scientific Publications, Lyon. pp 19-212, 1978.

Mirvish SS. Effects of vitamins C and E on N-nitroso compound formation, carcinogenesis and cancer. Cancer 58:1842-1850, 1986.

Bostick RM et al. Reduced risk of colon cancer with high intake of vitamin E: The Iowa Women's health Study. Cancer Research 53:4230-4237, 1993

Safety of Vitamin E
Bendich A et al. Safety of oral intake of vitamin E. American Journal of Clinical Nutrition 48:612-619, 1988.

Who Shouldn't Take Vitamin E
VERIS Vitamin E research Summary. February 1991.

Chapter 5: How Vitamin C Can Protect Your Health.

Smokers Deficient in Vitamin C
Murata A. Smoking and vitamin C. World Review of Nutrition and Dietetics 64:31-57, 1991.

Calder JH et al. Comparison of vitamin C in plasma and leukocytes of smokers and nonsmokers. Lancet i:556, 1963.

Brook M et al. Vitamin C concentration of plasma and leukocytes as related to smoking habits, age and sex of humans. American Journal of Clinical Nutrition 21:1254- 1258, 1968.

Bailey DA et al. Vitamin C supplementation related to physiological response to exercise in smoking and nonsmoking subjects. American Journal of Clinical Nutrition 23:905-912, 1970.

Burr ML et al. Plasma and leukocyte ascorbic acid levels in the elderly. American Journal of Clinical Nutrition 27:144- 131, 1974.

Albanese AA et al. An improved method for determination of leukocyte and plasma ascorbic acid of man with applications to studies on nutritional needs and effects of cigarette smoking. Nutrition Reports International 12:271-289, 1975.

Biersner RJ et al. Relationship of plasma vitamin C to the health and performance of submariners. Journal of Applied Nutrition 34:29-37, 1982.

Bazzarre TL. Effect of vitamin C supplementation among male smokers. Nutrition Reports International 33:711-720, 1986.

Basu J et al. Plasma reduced and total ascorbic acid in healthy women: effects of smoking and oral contraception. Contraception 39:85-93, 1989.

Elwood PC et al. Ascorbic acid and serum cholesterol. Lancet ii:1197, 1970.

Hoefel OS. Plasma vitamin C levels in smokers. International Journal Vitamin and Nutrition Research, supplement 16:127-137, 1977.

Chow CK et al. Lower levels of vitamin C and carotenes in plasma of cigarette smokers. Journal of American College of Nutrition. 5:305-312, 1986.

Keith RE et al. Effects of chronic cigarette smoking on vitamin C status, lung function, and resting and exercise cardiovascular metabolism in humans. Nutrition Reports International 21:907-912, 1980.

Keith RE et al. Ascorbic acid status of smoking and nonsmoking adolescent females. International Journal of Vitamin and Nutrition Research 56:363-366, 1986.

Pelletier O. Smoking and vitamin C levels in humans. American Journal of Clinical Nutrition 21:1259-1267, 1968.

Pelletier O. Vitamin C and tobacco. International Journal of Vitamin and Nutrition Research 16:147-169, 1977.

McClean HE et al. Vitamin C concentration in plasma and leukocytes of men related to age and smoking habit. New Zealand Medical Journal 83:226-229, 1976.

Murata A et al. Plasma and urine vitamin C levels in male smokers at periodic health examinations. Vitamins (Kyoto) 58:61-69, 1984.

Murata A et al. Lower levels of vitamin C in plasma and urine of Japanese male smokers. International Journal of Vitamin and Nutrition Research 31:184-189, 1989.

Schectman G et al. The influence of smoking on vitamin C status in adults. American Journal of Public Health 79:158- 162, 1989.

Tribble DL et al. Reduced plasma ascorbic acid concentrations in nonsmokers regularly exposed to environmental tobacco smoke. American Journal of Clinical Nutrition 58:886-890, 1993.

Vitamin C and Protection From Heart Disease
Gey KF et al. Plasma levels of antioxidant vitamins in relation to ischemic heart disease and cancer. American Journal of Clinical Nutrition 45:1368-1377, 1987.

Lehr H-A et al. Vitamin C prevents cigarette smoke-induced leukocyte aggregation and adhesion to endothelium in vivo. Proceedings of the National Academy of Sciences Vol 91, pp 7688-7692, 1994. Medical Sciences.

Vitamin C and Cancer Prevention
Block G. Vitamin C and cancer prevention: the epidemiologic evidence. American Journal of Clinical Nutrition 53:270S- 282S, 1991.

Block G. Human data on vitamin C in cancer prevention. In "Vitamins and Cancer Prevention", Pennington Center Nutrition Series vol 3, Louisiana State University Press, 1993.

References   123

Lung cancer
Fontham ETH et al. Dietary vitamins A and C and lung cancer in Louisiana. Cancer 62:2267-2273, 1988.

Koo LC. Dietary habits and lung cancer risk among Chinese females in Hong Kong who never smoked. Nutrition and Cancer 11:155-172, 1988.

Holst PA et al. For debate: pet birds as an independent risk factor for lung cancer. British Medical Journal 297:1319-1321, 1988.

Le Marchand L et al. Vegetable consumption and lung cancer risk: a population-based case-control study in Hawaii. Journal of the National Cancer Institute 81:1158-1164, 1989.

Kromhout D. Essential micronutrients in relation to carcinogenesis. American Journal of Clinical Nutrition 45:1361-1367, 1987.

Hinds MW et al. Dietary vitamin A, carotene, vitamin C and risk of lung cancer in Hawaii. American Journal of Epidemiology 119:227-237, 1984.

Kvale G et al Dietary habits and lung cancer risk. International Journal of Cancer 31:397-405, 1983.

Shekelle RB et al. Dietary vitamin A and risk of cancer in the Western Electric study. Lancet 2:1185-1190, 1981.

Byers TE et al. Dietary vitamin A and lung cancer risk: an analysis by histologic subtypes. American Journal of Epidemiology 120:769-776, 1984.

Byers TE et al. Diet and lung cancer: findings from the Western New York diet study. American Journal of Epidemiology 125:351-363, 1987.

Long-de W et al. Lung cancer, fruit, green salad and vitamin pills. China Medical Journal 98:206-210, 1985.

Bond GG et al. Dietary vitamin A and lung cancer: results of a case-control study among chemical workers. Nutrition and Cancer 9:109-121, 1987.

Mouth and throat cancer
Rossings MA et al. Diet and pharyngeal cancer. American Journal of Epidemiology 130:779 (abstract), 1989.

McGlaughlin JK et al. Dietary factors in oral and pharyngeal cancer. Journal of the National Cancer Institute 80:1237-1243, 1988.

Marshall J et al. Diet in the epidemiology of oral cancer. Nutrition and Cancer 3:145-149, 1982. Franco EL et al. Risk factors for oral cancer in Brazil: a case-control study. International Journal of Cancer 43:992-1000, 1989.

Wynder EL et al. A study of the etiological factors in cancer of the mouth. Cancer 10:1300-1321, 1957.

Notani PN et al. Role of diet in upper aerodigestive tract cancer. Nutrition and Cancer 10:103-113, 1987.

Graham S et al. Dietary factors in the epidemiology of cancer of the larynx. American Journal of Epidemiology 113:675-680, 1981.

Brown LM et al. Environmental factors and high risk of esophageal cancer among men in coastal South Carolina. Journal of the National Cancer Institute 80:1620-1625, 1988.

Tuyns AJ. Diet and esophageal cancer in Calvados (France). Nutrition and Cancer 9:81-92, 1987.

Zeigler RG et al. Esophageal cancer among black men in Washington DC, II: Role of nutrition. Journal of the National Cancer Institute 67:1199-1206, 1981.

Mettlin C et al. Diet and cancer of the esophagus. Nutrition and Cancer 2;143-147, 1980.

Cook-Mozaffari PJ et al. Esophageal cancer studies in the Caspian littoral of Iran: results of a case control study. British Journal of Cancer. 39:293-309, 1979.

Hirayama T et al. Naturally occurring carcinogens-mutagens and modulators of carcinogenesis. Tokyo: Japan Scientific Society Press, 359-380, 1979.

Bjelke E. Epidemiologic studies of cancer of the stomach, colon and rectum; with special emphasis on the role of diet. Vols 1-4. Doctoral dissertation, 1973. Ann Arbor MI: University Microfilms International, 1973.

Martinez I. Factors associated with cancer of the esophagus, mouth and pharynx in Puerto Rico. Journal of the National Cancer Institute 42:1069-1094, 1969.

Decarli A et al. Vitamin A and other dietary factors in the etiology of esophageal cancer. Nutrition and Cancer 10:29- 37, 1987.

Stomach cancer
Bjelke E. Case-control study of cancer of the stomach, colon and rectum. In "Oncology 1970: Being the Proceedings of the Tenth International Cancer Congress. Vol V. A. Environmental causes. B. Epidemiology and demography. C. Cancer education". Chicago: Yearbook Medical Publishers, Inc, 320-334, 1971.

Bjelke E. Epidemiology of colorectal cancer, with emphasis on diet. In "Human cancer. Its Characterization and treatment. Advances in tumor prevention, detection and characterization." Vol 5. Proceedings of the Eighth International Symposium on the Biological Characteristics of Human Tumors. Athens, May 8-11, 1979. Princeton: Excerpta Medica, 1980:158-174.

Correa P et al Dietary determinants of gastric cancer in south Louisiana inhabitants. Journal of the National Cancer Institute 73:645-654, 1985.

You W-C et al. Diet and high risk of stomach cancer in Shandong, China. Cancer Research 48:3518-3523, 1988.

LaVecchia C et al. A case-control study of diet and gastric cancer in northern Italy. International Journal of Cancer 40:484-489, 1987.

Risch HA et al. Dietary factors and the incidence of cancer of the stomach. American Journal of Epidemiology 122:947- 959, 1985.

Meinsma L. Nutrition and Cancer. Voeding 25:357-365, 1964. (in German).

Stahelin HB et al. Dietary risk factors for cancer in the Basel Study. Bibl Nutr Dieta 37:144-153, 1986.

Kono S et al. A case-control study of gastric cancer and diet in Northern Kyushu, Japan. Japanese Journal of Cancer Research 79:1067-1074, 1988.

Jedrychowski W et al. A case-control study of dietary factors and stomach cancer risk in Poland. International Journal of Cancer 37:837-842, 1986.

Trichopoulos D et al. Diet and cancer of the stomach: a case-control study in Greece. International Journal of Cancer 36:291-297, 1985.

Coggan D et al. Stomach cancer and food storage. Journal of the National Cancer Institute 81:1178-1182, 1989.

Cancers of the colon and rectum
Kune GA et al. The nutritional causes of colorectal cancer: an introduction to the Melbourne Study. Nutrition and Cancer 9:1-4, 1987.

Kune S et al. Case-control study of dietary etiological factors: the Melbourne colorectal cancer study. Nutrition and Cancer 9:21-42, 1987.

Tuyns AJ et al. Colorectal cancer and the intake of nutrients: oligosaccharides are a risk factor, fats are not. A case-control study in Belgium. Nutrition and Cancer 10:181-196, 1987.

Potter JD et al. Diet and cancer of the colon and rectum: a case-control study. Journal of the National Cancer Institute 76:557-569, 1986.

Heilbrun LK et al. Diet and colorectal cancer with specific reference to fiber intake. International Journal of Cancer 44:1-6, 1989.

La Vecchia C et al. A case-control study of diet and colo-rectal cancer in northern Italy. International Journal of Cancer 41:492-498, 1988.

Macquart-Moulin G et al. Case-control study on colorectal cancer and diet in Marseilles. International Journal of Cancer 38:183-191, 1986.

Jain M et al. A case-control study of diet and colo-rectal cancer. International Journal of Cancer 26:757-768, 1980.

Modan B et al. A note on the role of dietary retinol and carotene in human gastro-intestinal cancer. International Journal of Cancer 28:421-424, 1981.

Slattery ML et al. Diet and colon cancer: assessment of risk by fiber type and food source. Journal of the National Cancer Institute 80:1474-1480, 1988.

Haenszel W et al. Large-bowel cancer in Hawaiian Japanese. Journal of the National Cancer Institute 51:1765-1779, 1973.

Young TB et al. Case-control study of proximal and distal colon cancer and diet in Wisconsin. International Journal of Cancer 42:167-175, 1988.

Manousos O et al. Diet and colorectal cancer: a case-control study in Greece. International Journal of Cancer 32:1-5, 1983.

Cervical cancer
Marshall JR et al. Diet and smoking in the epidemiology of cancer of the cervix. Journal of the National Cancer Institute 70:847-851, 1983.

Wassertheil-Smoller S et al. Dietary vitamin C and uterine cervical dysplasia. American Journal of Epidemiology 114:714-724, 1981.

Brock KE et al. Nutrients in diet and plasma and risk of in situ cervical cancer. Journal of the National Cancer Institute 80:580-585, 1988.

Verreault R et al. A case-control study of diet and invasive cervical cancer. International Journal of Cancer 43:1050-1054, 1989.

Pancreatic cancer
Falk RT et al. Lifestyle risk factors for pancreatic cancer in Louisiana: a case-control study. American Journal of Epidemiology 128:324-336, 1988.

Norell SE et al. Diet and pancreatic cancer: a case-control study. American Journal of epidemiology 124:894-902, 1986.

Mack TM et al. Pancreas cancer and smoking, beverage consumption, and past medical history. Journal of the National Cancer Institute 76:49-60, 1986.

Gold EB et al. Diet and other risk factors for cancer of the pancreas. Cancer 55:460-467, 1985.

Mills PK et al.Dietary habits and past medical history as related to fatal pancreas cancer risk among Adventists. Cancer 61:2578-2585, 1988.

Breast cancer
Howe GR et al. Dietary factors and risk of breast cancer: combined analysis of 12 case-control studies. Journal of the National Cancer Institute 82:561-569, 1990.

Katsouyanni K et al. Risk of breast cancer among Greek women in relation to nutrient intake. Cancer 61:181-185, 1988.

Rohan TE et al. A population-based case-control study of diet and breast cancer in Australia. American Journal of Epidemiology 128:478-489, 1988.

La Vecchia C et al. Dietary factors and the risk of breast cancer. Nutrition and Cancer 10:205-214, 1987.

Brisson J et al. Diet, mammographic features of breast tissue, and breast cancer risk. American Journal of Epidemiology 130:14-24, 1989.

Toniolo P et al. Calorie-providing nutrients and risk of breast cancer. Journal of the National Cancer Institute 81:278-286, 1989.

Vitamin C and Cataract
Robertson JMcD et al. A possible role for vitamins C and E in cataract prevention. American Journal of Clinical Nutrition 53:346S-351S, 1991.

Jacques PF et al. Epidemiologic evidence of a role for the antioxidant vitamins and carotenoids in cataract prevention. American Journal of Clinical Nutrition 53:352S- 355S, 1991.

Vitamin C, Sperm Count and Fertility
Dawson EB et al. Effect of ascorbic acid supplementation on the sperm quality of smokers. Fertility and Sterility 58:8:1034-1039, 1992.

Fraga CG et al. Ascorbic acid protects against endogenous oxidative DNA damage in human sperm. Proceedings of the National Academy of Sciences 88:11003-11006, 1991.

Vitamin C and Toxic Metals
Sohler A et al. Blood lead levels in psychiatric outpatients reduced by zinc and vitamin C. Journal of Orthomolecular Psychiatry 6:272-276, 1977.

Vitamin C and Periodontal Disease (gum disease)
US Department of Health and Human Services (1986). Detection and prevention of periodontal disease in diabetes. NIH Publication no 86-1148.

Rivera-Hidaglo RF. Smoking and periodontal disease: a review of the literature. Journal Periodontology 57:617- 624, 1986.

Aurer-kozelji et al.The effect of ascorbic acid supplementation on periodontal tissue ultrastructure in subjects with progressive periodontitis. International Journal of Vitamin and Nutrition Research 52:333-341, 1982.

Buzina R et al. Increase of gingival hydroxyproline and proline by improvement of ascorbic acid status in man. International Journal of Vitamin and Nutrition Research 56:367-372, 1986

Leggott PJ et al. The effect of controlled ascorbic acid depletion and supplementation on periodontal health. Journal of Periodontology 57:480-485, 1986

How Much Vitamin C Do You Need
Kallner AB et al. On the requirements of ascorbic acid in man: steady state turnover and body pool in smokers. American Journal of Clinical Nutrition 34:1347-1355, 1981.

Schectman G et al. The influence of smoking on vitamin C status in adults. American Journal of Public Health 79:158- 162, 1989.

Pelletier O. Vitamin C status of cigarette smokers and nonsmokers. American Journal of Clinical Nutrition 23:520- 524, 1970.

Murata A et al. Lower levels of vitamin C in plasma and urine of Japanese male smokers. International Journal of Vitamin and Nutrition Research 31:184-189, 1989.

Safety of Vitamin C
Schmidt K-H et al. Urinary oxalate excretion after large intakes of ascorbic acid in man. American Journal of Clinical Nutrition 34:305-311, 1981.

Sutton JL et al. Effects of large doses of ascorbic acid in man on some nitrogenous components of urine. Human Nutrition, Applied Nutrition 37A:136-140, 1983.

Hoffer A. Ascorbic acid and kidney stones. Canadian Medical Association Journal 132:320, 1983.

Erden F et al. Effects of vitamin C intake on whole blood plasma, leukocyte and urine ascorbic acid and urine oxalic acid levels. Acta Vitaminologica et Enzymologica. 7:123- 130, 1985.

Singh PP et al. An investigation into the role of ascorbic acid in renal calculogenisis in albino rats. Journal of Urology 139:156-157, 1988.

Chapter 6: Other Vitamins and Minerals That can Help Smokers.

Preston AM. Cigarette smoking - nutritional implications. Progress in Food and Nutrition Science 15:183-217, 1991.

Vitamin B12
Department of Health and Human Services. Smoking and Health. A Report of the Surgeon General. Rockville MD., 1979.

Nakazawa Y et al. Serum folic acid levels and antipyrine clearance rates in smokers and nonsmokers. Drug and Alcohol Dependence. 11:201-208, 1983.

Linnell JC et al. Effects of smoking on metabolism and excretion of vitamin B12. British Medical Journal 2:215- 216, 1968.

Phillips CI et al. Vitamin B12 content of aqueous humor. Nature 217:67-68, 1968.

Wilson J et al. Metabolic inter-relationships between cyanide, thiocyanide, and vitamin B12 in smokers and nonsmokers. Clinical Science 31:1-7, 1966.

Wells DG et al. Thiocyanate metabolism in human vitamin B12 deficiency. British Medical Journal 4:588-590, 1972.

Heimberger DG et al. Improvement in bronchial squamous metaplasia in smokers treated with folate and vitamin B12. Journal of the American Medical Association 259:10; 1525- 1530, 1988.

Dastur DK et al. Effect of vegetarianism and smoking on vitamin B12, thiocyanate, and folate levels in the blood of normal subjects. British Medical Journal 3:260-263, 1972.

Folic Acid
Piyathilake CJ et al. Local and synthetic effects of cigarette smoking on folate and vitamin B12. American Journal of Clinical Nutrition 60:559-566, 1994.

Ortega RM et al. Influence of smoking on folate intake and blood folate concentrations in a group of elderly spanish men. Journal of the American College of Nutrition 13:1:68- 72, 1994.

US Dept of Health and Human Services, Centers for Disease Control, Morbidity and Mortality Weekly Report Vol 41/No RR-14, 11 September 1992.

Witter FR et al. Folate, carotene and smoking. American Journal of Obstetrics and Gynecology 144:857, 1982.

Chisholm IA. Serum cobalamin and folate in optic neuropathy associated with tobacco smoking. Canadian Journal of Opthalmology 13:105-109, 1978.

Heimberger DG et al. Localized folic acid deficiency and bronchial metaplasia in smokers. Hypothesis and preliminary report. Nutrition International 3:54-60, 1987.

Vitamin B6
Serfontein WJ et al. Depressed plasma pyridoxal 5 phosphate levels in tobacco-smoking men. Atherosclerosis 59:341-346, 1986.

Vermaak WJH et al. Vitamin B6 nutrition status and cigarette smoking. American Journal of Clinical Nutrition 51:1058-1061, 1990.

Selenium
Diplock AT. Trace elements in human health with special reference to selenium. American Journal of Clinical Nutrition 45:1313-1322, 1987.

Chapter 7: The Fruit and Vegetable Connection.

Serdula MK et al. Fruit and vegetable intake among adults in 16 states: Results of a brief telephone survey. American Journal of Public Health 85:No2:236-239, 1995.

Five a Day - for Better Health. Eat more fruit and vegetables. U.S. Department of Health and Human Services brochure. NIH publication no 92-3248, 1991.

Five a Day - for Better Health. Eat more salads for better health. U.S. Department of Health and Human Services brochure. NIH publication no 91-3250, 1992.

Five a Day - for Better Health. Easy entertaining with fruits and vegetables for better health. U.S. Department of Health and Human Services brochure. NIH publication no 92-3249, 1992.

Five a Day - for Better Health. Fast and easy. Fruits and vegetables for busy people. U.S. Department of Health and Human Services brochure. NIH publication no 92-3247, 1992.

Chapter 8: Other Health Protection Measures for Smokers.

Tea drinking

Chisaka T et al. The effect of crude drugs on experimental hypercholesteremia: mode of action of epigallocatechin gallate in tea leaves. Chemical and Pharmaceutical Bulletin (Tokyo) 36:227-233, 1988.

Fujita Y et al. Inhibitory effect of epigallocatechin gallate on carcinogenesis with N-ethyl-N'-nitro-N- nitrosoguanidine in mouse duodenum. Japanese Journal of Cancer Research 80:503-505, 1989.

Fujiki H et al New antitumor promoters: epigallocatechin gallate and sarcophytols A and B. Basic Life Sciences 52:205-212,1990.

Fijiki H. epigallocatechin gallate (EGCG), a cancer preventive agent. Fourth Chemical Congress of North America. New York: American Chemical Society, 1991.

Yang C et al. Protection against stomach, lung and esophageal carcinogenesis by green tea. Fourth Chemical Congress of North America. New York: American Chemical Society, 1991.

Chung P et al. Protection against tobacco-specific nitrosamine-induced lung tumorigenesis by green tea and its components. Fourth Chemical Congress of North America. New York: American Chemical Society, 1991.

Weisburger JH. Tea antioxidants and health. In "Handbook of Antioxidants", Cadenas & Packer (eds), Marcel Dekker Inc, NY, 1995.

Hensrud DD et al. Antioxidant status, fatty acids and cardiovascular disease. Nutrition 10:172-175, 1994.

Stensvold I et al. Tea consumption. Relationship to cholesterol, blood pressure, and coronary and total mortality. Preventive Medicine 21:546-553, 1992.

Green MS et al. Association of serum lipoproteins and health-related habits with coffee and tea consumption in free living subjects examined in the Israeli CORDIS study. Preventive Medicine 21:532-545, 1992.

Kono S et al. Green tea consumption and serum lipid profiles: A cross-sectional study in Northern Kyushu, Japan. Preventive Medicine 21:526-531, 1992.

Eating Fish May Protect Smoker's Lungs

Eyal S et al. Dietary n-3 polyunsaturated fatty acids and smoking-related chronic obstructive pulmonary disease. New England Journal of Medicine 331:228-233, 1994.

Schwartz J et al. Dietary factors and their relation to respiratory symptoms: the Second National Health and Nutrition Examination Survey. American Journal of Epidemiology 132:67-76, 1990.

Organization for Economic Co-operation and Development. Food consumption statistics: 1964-1978. Paris OECD, 1981.

Comstock GW et al. Respiratory findings and urban living. Archives of Environmental Health 27:143-150, 1973.

Aoki M. Epidemiology of chronic airways diseases in Japan. Chest 96:343S-349S (Suppl), 1989.

Chapter 9: The "quit smoking" Option.

Ashton H et al. Smoking, Psychology & Pharmacology, Tavistock Publications, London, 1982.

Schwartz JL. Smoking cessation methods: the United States and Canada. US Dept of Health and Human Services

Reducing the health consequences of smoking: 25 years of progress, a report of the Surgeon General, 1989. US Dept of Health and Human Services.

Appendix
Mail-order Vitamin Suppliers

For those readers who prefer to shop by mail or don't have a convenient local supplier, a list of companies who sell vitamins, minerals, green tea, etc by mail is given below. You can call, FAX or write for a catalog.

Nutrition Headquarters
One Nutrition Plaza
Carbondale
IL 62901
TEL 800 851 3551
FAX 618 529 4553

Bronson
1945 Craig Rd, PO 46903
St Louis
MO 63146-6903
TEL 800 235 3200
FAX 314 469 5741

Lee Nutrition
290 Main St
Cambridge
MA 02124
TEL 800 272 2745
FAX 617 661 6259

Freeda Vitamins
36 E 41st St
New York
NY 10017
TEL 800 777 3737
FAX 212 685 7297

Barth Vitamins
865 Merrick Ave
Westbury
NY 11590
TEL 800 645 2328
FAX 305 978 9097

Hillestad International Inc
AV178 US Hwy 51 N
Woodruff
WI 54568
TEL 800 535 7742
FAX 715 358 7812

Beyond A Century
HC76, Box 200
Geeenville
ME 04441
TEL 800 777 1324
FAX 207 695 2492

L & H Vitamins Inc
37-10 Cresent St
Long Island City
NY 11101
TEL 800 221 1152
FAX 718 361 1437

Vitamin Specialities Co
8200 Ogontz Ave
Wyncote
PA 19095
TEL 800 365 8482
FAX 215 885 1310

Puritan's Pride
1233 Montauk Highway,
PO Box 9001
Oakdale
NY 11769-9001
TEL 800 645 1030
FAX 516 471 5693

RVP Health Savings
Center
855 Merrick Ave
Westbury
NY 11590-6620
TEL 800 645 2978

SDV Vitamins
PO Box 23030
Oakland Park
FL 33307
TEL 800 535 7095
FAX 800 373 8329

Shelby Health Systems
342 Wolverine Way
Sparks
NV 89431-5728
TEL 800 490 8555
FAX 708 342 7477

Star Professional Pharma-
ceuticals
1500 New Horizons Blvd
Amityville
NY 11701
TEL 800 274 6400
FAX 800 433 3291

Vitamin Discount
Connection
35 North 8th St
PO Box 1431
Indiana
PA 15701
TEL 800 848 2990
FAX 412 349 3711

Vitamin Shoppe
4700 Westside Ave
North Bregen
NJ 07047
TEL 800 223 1216
FAX 201 866 9513

Glossary

Aggregation: the massing or clumping of materials together.

Alpha carotene: a member of the carotene family of compounds, found in pumpkin and carrots.

Alveolar fluid: fluid coating found on the inner surface of the lungs.

Antioxidant: any substance which prevents oxidation.

Arthritis: a disease characterized by inflammation of, and pain in the joints.

Ascorbic acid: vitamin C.

Bacteria: single-celled microorganisms.

Beriberi: a form of malnutrition due to deficiency of vitamin B1.

Beta carotene: the most commonly known member of the carotene family of compounds.

Beta cryptoxanthin: a little known member of the carotene family of compounds, found in papaya and oranges.

Bronchitis: inflammation of the air passages of the lungs.

Cancer: a disease characterized by a disorder of cell growth.

Carotenes: a group of over 600 naturally occurring substances which give many fruits and vegetables their yellow or orange/red coloring.

Carotenoids: carotenes.

Cataract: the progressive clouding of the lens of the eye leading eventually to blindness.

Cervical: of the neck of the womb.

Cervix: the neck of the womb.

Chelation: process where a substance combines with a metal, commonly used in cases of metal poisoning.

Chlorophyll: the green coloring matter found in leaves and plants essential to the production of carbohydrates by photosynthesis.

Cholesterol: a fat-like substance, the main component of deposits in the lining of arteries.

Chronic: persisting for a long time.

Colitis: inflammation of the colon.

Collagen: a fibrous structural protein, the principal component of skin, tendon, bone, cartilage and other connective tissue.

Colon: the lower bowel extending to the rectum.

d-alpha-tocopherol: the principal member of the vitamin E family of substances.

Degenerative: that which leads to deterioration.

DNA: deoxyribonucleic acid, the self-replicating substance of genes, the genetic blueprint.

Dysplasia: alteration in size, shape and organization of cells.

Emphysema: a disease of the lungs where bronchioles become plugged with mucus.

Endrometrial: of the lining of the uterus.

Enzymes: any protein which promotes chemical change.

Epidemiology: the study of the relationships of the various factors determining the frequency and distribution of diseases.

Esophagus: the passage extending from the pharynx to the stomach.

FDA: Food and Drug Administration.

Folate: folic acid.

Folic acid: a member of the B vitamin group, found in green plants.

Food and Drug Administration: an arm of the Federal government charged with regulating new drugs entering the market place, ensuring the quality of all manufactured drugs and protecting the population from unsafe medicines.

Food and Nutrition Board: a branch of the National Research Council.

Free Radical: dangerous molecules in our bodies that can damage or destroy cells.

Gastrointestinal: of the stomach and intestine.

Gene: one of the biologic units of heredity.

Genetic: of the branch of biology dealing with heredity and the laws governing it.

Gram: the basic unit of weight of the metric system, being equivalent to approximately one twenty-eighth of an ounce, written in abbreviated form "g".

Gynecology: medicine and surgery of the female reproductive system.

Immune system: the body's defense mechanism which combats disease or foreign microbes.

Infection: invasion and multiplication of disease-causing microorganisms in body tissue.

Infectious: caused by or capable of being communicated by infection.

Inflammatory: causing inflammation.

Inflammation: a defensive response to injury or irritation.

Inherited: having characters or qualities acquired by transmission from parent to offspring.

IU: abbreviation of International Unit. A measure of the amount of active ingredient.

Larynx: the voice-box at the entrance to the windpipe in the front of the neck.

Lesion: disturbance of the structure or function of a part of the body, such as a wound, abscess, ulcer, tumor or other tissue damage.

Leukocyte: white blood cells whose main function is to protect the body against microorganisms causing disease.

Leukoplakia: small white patches on the mucus membrane, usually in the mouth, often the result of pipe smoking or the chewing of tobacco. May lead to cancer.

Lutein: a member of the carotene family of compounds, found in green leafy vegetables.

Lycopene: a member of the carotene family of compounds, found in tomatoes and guava.

Manganese: a chemical element, occurs in very small amounts in body tissue.

Microbe: a living creature too small to be seen with the naked eye. Certain types can cause disease by infection.

Microgram: one millionth of one gram, 1/1,000,000 gram, written in abbreviated form as "mcg".

Milligram: one thousandth of one gram, 1/1,000 gram, written in abbreviated form as "mg".

Mineral: any naturally occuring non-organic solid substance. There are 19 or more minerals in the composition of the body, and at least 13 of these are essential to health.

Molecule: the smallest complete unit of a substance.

National Academy of Sciences: private honorary organization dedicated to the furtherance of science and engineering. Founded by an act of Congress to serve as official advisor to the federal government on scientific and technical matters.

Nitrosamine: cancer-causing substances found in some foods, produced in the body by reactions with certain foods and by the action of cigarette smoke components.

Nutrient: a nourishing substance, food or component of food.

Nutrition: the processes involved in taking in nutrients and utilizing them.

Obstetrics: the branch of medicine dealing with pregnancy and childbirth.

Omega-3 fatty acids: polyunsaturated fats whose major source in human foods is fish.

Optimum: the best or most favorable degree or condition.

Oral: of the mouth.

Oxidation: process of cell metabolism resulting in the release of energy.

Pancreas: a large gland located behind the stomach involved in the digestive process.

Periodontal: of the tissues surrounding and supporting the teeth.

Pharynx: the throat.

Platelet: the smallest of the solid particles suspended in the blood.

Polyunsaturated: having more than one double bond in its hydrocarbon chain.

Precancerous: a condition tending to lead to cancer.

Protein: essential ingredients of all living matter. They make up about 12% of the weight of the human body (water is 70% and fat 15%)

Pro-vitamin: a substance the body can convert to a vitamin.

Recommended Dietary Allowance: the level of intake of an essential nutrients judged by the Food and Nutrition Board to be adequate to meet the known nutrient needs of practically all healthy persons.

RDA: Recommended Dietary Allowance.

Rectum: the last few inches of the large intestine terminating in the anal canal.

Rheumatoid arthritis: a chronic disease with inflammatory changes throughout the body's connective tissues especially the joints.

Rickets: defective growth of bone due to lack of vitamin D.

Scurvy: a defect of the substance that binds cells together, especially connective tissue and blood vessels, due to lack of vitamin C.

Selenium: a chemical element, and essential nutrient.

Serum: clear fluid that remains after the solid elements have been separated from blood.

Singlet oxygen molecule: a highly reactive molecule produced in the body by oxidation. Generates large numbers of free radicals.

Stroke: rupture or blockage of a blood vessel in the brain, depriving parts of the brain of blood supply.

Tissue: a group of similarly specialized cells that together perform certain special functions.

Tocopherols: family of substances from which vitamin E is derived.

Toxic: poisonous.

Ulcerative colitis: recurrent ulceration of the colon.

Ultraviolet light: part of the spectrum of light invisible to the human eye.

Vaccine: a suspension of modified or killed microorganisms given to prevent or treat infectious diseases.

Virus: the smallest microbe, most are too small to be seen with an ordinary microscope.

Vitamin: any organic substance found in foods and essential in small quantities for growth or health.

Vitamin A: manufactured in man and animals from carotenes and obtained directly from animal products such as liver, eggs, whole milk, cream and cheese. Essential for night vision.

Zeaxanthin: a member of the carotene family of compounds, found in green leafy vegetables.

Zinc: a chemical element, and essential nutrient.

Index

About the Author

Alistair Moodie was born in Ayr, a small county town on the west coast of Scotland. His father, a country veterinarian much in the mold of James Herriot of "All Creatures Great and Small" fame, taught him from an early age the value of common sense and an independent mind. He graduated with a Batchelor of Science degree from Heriot-Watt University Edinburgh, Scotland in 1971.

Despite the strong influence of non-smoking parents, Moodie took up the habit in his early teens and continued to smoke, more or less continuously for nearly twenty-five years, eventually "quitting for good" at age 38. A family history of lung complaints and his father's early death from heart disease drove him to search for ways to reduce the health risks.

He lives in Maryland with his wife Margaret and two-year-old daughter Fiona.

Do you have friends or loved ones who smoke ?

Help them protect their health, give them a copy of this book as a gift ! Use the order form below:

ORDER FORM
Cut out or photocopy this page and fill in the details below:

Please send _____ copies of THE SMOKER'S GUIDE TO VITAMINS AND HEALTH
Books are $9.95 each plus $2.00 per book shipping and handling.
Total enclosed $_____
Make checks or money order payable to:
Vanguard Books.

Delivery address:
Please print clearly.

Name _____

Address _____

City _____

State _____   Zip _____

Send this order form together with your check or money order for the above amount to:

> Vanguard Books
> PO Box 4028
> Crofton
> MD 21114

If you require bulk orders of this book, please write for discount schedule.